Total Health

LDS Perspective

Chris Fife
© 12/30/14

Table of Contents

Introduction

Achieving and maintaining good health is something we all struggle to do throughout our lives. For some it can be a great mystery or difficult journey. The best of athletes struggle to be healthy. It is a lifelong pursuit to be healthy.

This book is a guideline for being healthy. It cannot replace common sense, hard work, and diligence in developing healthy habits. It can help the reader lay a foundation for a healthy life.

The book takes an LDS perspective. This means that members of the Church of Jesus Christ of Latter-day Saints will be familiar with the scriptural references and the Word of Wisdom as it relates to health. Members are no strangers to the healthy practices of the church, however there are some incites for members to think about when it comes to their health.

Total Health examines several aspects of health such as spiritual health, social health, and financial health which are not normally covered in a health related book. It is important to note that in order to enjoy overall health you need to look at these other areas. It is difficult at best to be healthy when your spiritual or social health is suffering. The book takes a holistic approach to health. It also examines pitfalls we face when it comes to health.

This book does not go into a fad diet or a cure all exercise routine. These things are left up to the reader to develop their own personal healthy habits. The book gives suggestions and ideas for the reader to start their own routines and diets.

Chapter One: Health in America

"The devil has put a penalty on all things we enjoy in life. Either we suffer in health or we suffer in soul or we get fat." Albert Einstein.

According to the CDC there is roughly 2,437,163 people dying in the United States each year, and of those about 48% are dying from Heart Disease and Cancer. The two main causes of deaths in America come from smoking and obesity which is the result of eating too much and lack of physical activity. In the top ten much of the deaths in America were caused by smoking and obesity and these two things cost over a hundred billion dollars a year. Our lives are filled with things about health and the news is constantly giving stories about health.

One of the main political debates has been for many years health care and what America needs to do to help people have adequate health care. Many of us question the cost and reliability of our health care system, and the manipulation of the food industry to get people to buy unhealthy foods. With over a million deaths a year we spend a lot of time and money on research, healthy promotions, and stress over something that should be as simple as just taking care of ourselves. Only it becomes much more complicated than that.

Surprisingly suicide is number 10 in deaths in America with over 30,000 a year. So there is also an increasing alarm when it comes to stress in our lives and the ability to cope with such stress. In part we have a growing concern when it comes to health issues in America.

Compared to other countries the World Health Organization has ranked the United States as 37th in the world for quality health care. France is number one, and Japan is number 10 in the world. Also when it comes to life expectancy the United States is 29th with Japan being number one. So the United States is not the healthiest place to live, and considering the wealth and the advancements in medicine in the United States you would think that the United States would be a lot higher in the rankings, but most European countries are higher than the United States as well as some Latin American countries like Chile.

The lowest countries on the rankings on the World Health Organization ranking system are many African countries and other countries in the world that have high poverty rates, and have suffered war, or other huge challenges in health care. The bottom line is that while in many other countries their low health status is a systematic political mess, the United States tends to not be the lack of technology and advancements in health, it tends to be more of an overall lack of physical, mental, and spiritual health related to pride and wealth.

In America we are not just unhealthy because we eat too much and have poor health habits. It is that we spend most of our time in front of television screens, computer screens, or phone screens being absorbed by media propaganda that is causing a lot of mixed, confusing, and often misunderstood health information and messages.

On one hand we all know that it is not healthy to smoke, yet we allow the sale and distribution of tobacco products in the United States, and until just since the massive lawsuit against the tobacco industry we allowed tobacco advertisements that mislead the public and targeted children. Since the restriction of tobacco advertisements and the aggressive campaign to stop smoking and laws preventing people in many states from smoking in public buildings and parks, the amount of people who smoke has gone down, as well as the deaths associated with smoking.

We know that is has been effective to aggressively attack the tobacco companies, yet we are still falling short when it comes to the food industry with all of the advertisements that are shown including alcohol commercials. The food industry is a billion dollar industry that is controlled by a handful of giant companies who dictate what is made and sold to the American people and sent to other countries around the world. Deaths related to food poisoning, as well as obesity continue to go up each year in part to the greed of the food companies and the lack of responsibility to produce healthy products. Just like with the tobacco companies, fast food companies also target children with Happy Meals, and toys. The restaurants often advertise children's movies with promotional toys and posters to lure children into the restaurant so that they could get the toy about the movie they want to go see or have already seen. It isn't any wonder that there are more obese children every year.

According to the CDC every state has over 20% of their population as being obese which is being over 30 on the BMI (Body Mass Index) which shows a scale of how much a person should weigh according to their height. For many this means being 20 to 30 pounds overweight or more according to the BMI. This means that a person who is five feet six inches tall would be overweight if they weighed over 150 pounds and obese at 180 pounds. A third of all adults are obese which is at 35.7% and children the ages of (2-19) at 17% at about 12.5 million children in the United States.

It is expected that adults have higher incidents of obesity than children because the metabolism in adults slows and activity level decreases and food consumption increases. But still to have 12.5 million children obese that means that they will be obese as adults and probably for the rest of their lives with all of the medical conditions associated with it.

There are more cases of children dying from a heart attack, cancer, and other disease that were generally reserved for adults. More children are having type 2 diabetes, and poor health due to their lifestyle and being obese. It is crazy to think that there are so many children with health problems, and the cost of health care is rising with each generation. Yet we only teach a half a year of health in high school, and only require a year of physical education and in some states the year of physical education can be done online or be exempted. Children are more inclined to just text their friends, play video games, and watch television than to do physical play. Increasingly our society is getting more away from physical activity and eating more.

There have been some positive changes in the way things are done. But this has only been after law suits and the World Health Organization giving suggestions that things are slowly starting to change, but some of this seems more temporary than a long term solution. I no longer hear a lot of talk about HIV, because not as many people die from it each year in the United States and so the aggressive education of the public is almost gone. The same thing has happened to food. One moment schools are serving healthy snacks in their vending machines the next the unhealthy stuff is back.

We still have not aggressively targeted getting people active and responsible eaters. It is because of our culture which is food oriented and physically reserved for athletes and fitness fanatics. Only about 10 percent of the population in the United States exercises on a daily basis, which is recommended by experts. Many restaurants serve portion sizes that can feed three adults. Americans feel that they deserve a large meal, and when they pay the money they expect a lot for their money.

Everything is centered around food. All holidays have food involved in it, and not healthy food but sugary candy and fattening foods. Just think about Halloween, Thanksgiving, Christmas, Valentine's Day, and Easter. You just have to go into any store around these holidays and there are entire rows filled with candy and junk foods. Some stores stock up a month or more before the holiday with such foods, and then have sales up to a month later to get rid of it. This means that Americans eat this holiday junk over half the year.

Then just think of all of the family celebrations, the work related parties, the church functions all of which contain food. We then start to associate food with having a good time. Think of the last time you celebrated something by not eating food, or just having healthy food. I remember going over to my grandparent's house and eating candy and ice cream. I often wonder if it was the candy and ice cream that made me more excited about seeing my grandparents than just seeing my grandparents because I loved them. We use food as a bribe in school, home, community, and even at church. I remember for a primary celebration for reading scriptures they had a pizza party.

I do not think there is anything wrong with having celebrations and eating candy and ice cream, but it is the quantity of it that matters, and how we associate it in our lives. If we think of food as a happy drug then we will indulge every time we feel sad and depressed. We need food to survive, but it can be addictive to the point that we will binge on food until it makes us sick.

The same thing goes with physical fitness, there are times when we might play games at family reunions along with all of the food and desserts we eat. We might play basketball or soccer at a social or a party, but generally there are only a few who are playing and it is not as a tradition or comfort to go play something as it is to just sit and eat. There are some communities, families, and even the church that promotes physical activity, but it is still far too less than it should be and we tend to have a stigmatism of running around and getting sweaty. Then there is the injuries associated with sports and physical activity that many people shy away from. Plus there is a social association with competition when it comes to physical activity. Many people get it in their mind that if they exercise they have to compete against someone or something like trying to lose weight.

It is only those who exercise because they enjoy it and think it is fun making it part of their life who are able to maintain a healthy lifestyle and weight. But how many people think exercise is fun and they would want to do it at least twenty minutes a day for the rest of their life taking only Sunday off with an occasional vacation. Only one out of ten Americans feel this way.

Then there is the stress we have in our lives and the moral degeneration of society. With the invention and proliferation of electronics and technology stress has increased dramatically in people's lives. Maybe you can remember a time in your life when you wanted to relax and not have anyone bother you including getting telephone calls. But now not only do we have telephones at home we carry them with us 24 hours a day seven days a week and feel that we are naked without them and unable to function properly.

People no longer wear watches, or carry cameras because they have them in their phones. With the technology, people can text, and talk to people from all over the world. They can check email messages, send email, watch videos, take pictures, listen to music, surf the internet, and do a variety of others things including playing video games. With all of this in your pocket why do you need to do anything else but spend the day with your cell phone. I wonder how many people if asked honestly would say that their cell phone was their best friend and they spent more time with it than their family, friends, and co-workers.

There are now evidence about how destructive cell phones and technology can be to a person's health when they become addictive and cannot do anything else but spend time on their cell phones or on the internet playing games. There are clinics to help people with these types of addictions.

It isn't any wonder why there are over 30,000 people in the United States who commit suicide every year, because of the stress they have put into their lives and the degenerative effects on our society in regards to morality and spirituality. Instead of putting their faith in God, and living a righteous life many people put their trust in money and things. Many people walk around without a sense of identity and have to get tattoos in order to indentify who they are. It becomes an odd relationship with the materialistic world.

Seeing the teenagers now with their tattoos, piercings, and gang related culture you can see just how far we have gone in our society. Some walk around like porcupines with all of the spikes they have coming from their face. Any rational person would see this as not normal behavior, yet teens see it as the new thing to do, and the more crazy they look the better. Only by doing such things they not only permanently alter their appearance they alter their mental and emotional state as well.

Instead of finding ways to help the rising generation to become lifelong learners and seek out fulfilling their dreams, we have built up a standard of competition, restrictions, and raising the bar on qualifications for everything. The government has said that they have to hold schools accountable for teaching children, and so they are coming up with more things to teach children. It seems like every year they require teachers to teach more material to children and then test the children to see how well the school has done, and instead of sticking with a program that works and working with children to master all of the skills and learn the material. The people in charge of the schools says that things are not working so they have to teach the children more things and then test them again.

There then becomes a dangerous cycle of cramming information and skills into children hoping that they will be able to master the skills and be ready for the next barrage of skills the next year. This means that many of the children are being left behind, because they cannot keep up with what is being taught, and there is nothing in place to need the child's needs, and then when the child is having trouble that is noticeable they pull the child out and tutor them, but then the child still is behind the rest of the students and will remain behind the rest of his years in school struggling to just survive. Some of these children simply give up and end up dropping out of school, others manage to be able to graduate from high school, but lack the skills to do anything, and thus have a hard time getting jobs and having relationships.

All of this means that stress and pressures to be successful are increasing each year, and not gradually, but exponentially to the point that the stress level of our children will be over a hundred times higher than when we went through school. Some would say it is good for them and that children need to learn more than they have in the past, and it is good to push them and they can only become better if they are in a competition mode. Only when the suicide rise and more and more children have health problems due to stress they might finally decide that they need to do things differently.

Obesity is rapidly becoming the number one cause of death and health related illness in America, but it is often the pressure and stress of life that is causing children and adults to binge eat in order to relieve their stress. Food contains chemicals that will release endorphins and other pleasure hormones into our brain and our bodies. Increased stress will also weaken the immune system thus causing children to have more allergies, and many other illnesses including cancer and heart disease. It might be cigarette smoking and over eating as the main causes of death and illness in the United States, but it is stress that is causing people to smoke and over eat.

Many people including children are slowly killing themselves because they have given up on life and all of the pressures that are involved in life. They might not be consciously thinking about committing suicide, but by eating too much, smoking, doing drugs, and having other risky behavior they are sending a message that they do not care about life anymore and they want to die.

Mental health is just as important as physical health. Millions of people every year suffer from some sort of mental illness. At one point in everyone's life they have suffered a mental illness. It could have been depression, sadness, or a sudden burst of anger or some sort of mental outburst because of a stressor. The brain is the command center for the entire body and so when it is affected in some sort of way it affects the rest of the body. It could come in the form of a headache, or exhaustion.

All of our physical actions are the results of our thoughts and emotions. We receive environmental stimulus through our senses and that stimulus goes to the brain in less than a micro second and converts it to thoughts, emotions, and ideas in the brain which compels us to act in a certain way. So if we receive negative stimulus like someone screaming at us calling us names then that will go back to the brain and cause us to get angry or withdraw and absorb the insults. In any cause our thoughts and emotions will affect our physical health as well.

Spiritual health is even more important that both mental and physical, because it is what keeps us together. If our spirit suffers then our mind and body will suffer as well. People who have lost hope and faith in themselves and in God tend to do destructive behaviors and have some sort of mental illness which in turns affects their physical health. Even faithful members of the church may suffer from spiritual decline from time to time. It is just as important to keep out spirits healthy as it is with our minds and bodies.

We will wash our hands and keep out bodies clean in order to stay off infection and disease, yet we often overlook the cleansing of our spirits from sin and wickedness. We have to cleanse our spirits as often as we clean our bodies. Once our spirits weaken they are susceptible to even greater darkness in our lives. In society instead of making spirituality a major part of our lives it is more of out of convenience that many people worship where they will attend church only when they feel like it or when it is convenient to them which means that they attend church once or twice a year generally around Christmas and Easter. They believe in God, only they do not believe that they have to put forth any effort in being religious, and think that they just have to not hurt someone and break laws in order to have a healthy spirit, and that those who are wicked are only the ones who kill, and rape.

Our society has rationalized such behavior as homosexuality, immorality, immodesty, and riotous living as being okay. It is almost as if there is a false sense of right and wrong. The extremes of violence and injury of other people is wrong, but if it doesn't hurt others, or is not perceived to harm others then it is okay. Students believe it is okay to cheat on tests, and to lie to friends. Many people believe it is okay to be immoral just so long as others are willing to be immoral as well.

Those who do commit sin will immediately start to rationalize what they had done was not bad. They will feel uncomfortable going to church because they will feel guilty for what they have done, and then they will start withdrawing from things that are important in their life like family, friends, the church, prayer, and reading the scriptures because those things only make them feel even more guilty for the things they have done. They will go to places and associate with people who are doing the same types of things in order to further rationalize what they are doing because other people are doing it as well and then all of them can discuss back and forth rationalizing what they have done feeling more comfortable that others are doing it as well.

When it comes to health it is a lot more complex than just eating a healthy diet, and exercising. There are a lot of factors involved with health that are often neglected in health books and are not always looked at as an influence on health. When we look at health we often look at the physical side of health, and sometimes the mental side as well. Some will include spiritual health, but often look at it in terms of a general ideal, or even more of an Eastern spiritual context like with Buddhism or Hinduism. It might also be discussed as more of a moral or high ideal way of living instead of something that is part of us with our souls.

Health is part of life that we cannot get around. It is always there and constantly remind us about it when we get aches and pains or get violently sick. It is these times when we are sick that we are reminded of our health and we make a promise to ourselves that we will eat better, exercise more frequently, and start living healthier lives. Only we get better and start to live healthier only to become more complacent when our lives become more complicated or busy and the first thing to go is the eating right and the exercise.

Most people go through these ups and downs when it comes to healthy living which allows for us to have a roller coaster relationship with healthy living and unhealthy consequences. Just like in the Book of Mormon when the Nephites became prosperous from their righteous living, then they start to be proud and think that it is okay to let their guard down and they start up being evil again. Then because of their evil ways they are cursed with all manner of illness and afflictions. Then they are humble and return

14

back to the Lord, and then they start living righteous lives again. The Nephites then start to become prosperous again and then wicked, and continue the cycle.

It is important not to have the roller coaster relationship with health in your life. You can save a lot of money, be happier, and healthier if you make taking care of your health part of your lifestyle. Just think about living a life without getting sick and free from pain, being happy all of the time and rejoicing in the Lord. Think how life would be if you could be able to have a comfortable where you are happy and enjoy family and friends. You would be able to go out and play with your children and grandchildren. You would be able to climb mountains, run in marathons, and do all those things you ever wanted to do.

Even those who are unhealthy will be able to significantly improve their health through starting to change their lifestyles. Imagine being able to do things you have always wanted to do like hiking, mountain biking, or just being able to walk to the park with your children. Life is filled with opportunities and wonderful experiences, but if you are unhealthy those opportunities and experiences are limited at best. The quality of life diminishes dramatically when health is diminished.

Health Care

I have briefly talked about health care and how the United States is ranked very low among industrialized countries. It seems that the mentality of health care in the United States is twofold do not do anything about health until it is in jeopardy and then treat it, and the other is to get medicine for every ailment you might have. Treatment is the main focus of medicine these days. People do what they want, eat what they want, and allow their health to deteriorate until they start to have problems and then they go see a doctor who suggests surgery or medications.

Surgery is invasive and will end up with further complications thus requiring more surgery or medicine. Medicines these days are expensive and cause further side effects and complications which requires more medications and more doctor visits. Once a person gets into the system then they are bound to it through all of these things that lead to other things.

Many people also tend to abuse both prescription medications and over the counter medications. If someone had a headache they take a pain medication, if they have aches and pains from gardening they take medications, if they get a cold or the flue they take medications. We live in a society that is filled with drug dealers and drug users and we are paying the price with high medical costs and poor health. Then there are the people who when they first get sick they run to the doctor's office to get medicine to take care of their illness. Then they do the same with their children, and the children learn that when they get sick they need to go to the doctor.

The reality of all of this is that because of American obsession to go to the doctor when getting sick and taking medications when getting sick the costs of medical care continues to increase and the quality of health and the health care system goes down. The truth is that most minor illnesses and aches go away without medical treatment and medicines. The common cold lasts about a week regardless of if you take medicine, see the doctor, or just stay home get rest and have chicken noodle soup. The difference is that if you take care of your cold yourself it is a lot less money involved, you become less dependent on doctors, your body is healthier for it because it is not taking in toxic medicine to suppress some of the cold symptoms.

There is no cure for the common cold, and many flu viruses even if you get a vaccination there are dozens of viruses that you could get that are not affected by the vaccination. The medicines taken for colds only mask the symptoms and may even interfere with the body's natural ability to fight the cold. So by taking medicines to get over the cold you might be prolonging having it. There are several things you can do to help you get rid of a cold and relieve the symptoms. These will be discussed in a later chapter.

When someone in America gets sick and they see a doctor, the doctor does some basic tests and an examination of the patient and then prescribes a medication. If it happens to be something that is internal or a physical injury then surgery might be an option. Very few doctors offer alternatives to meds or surgery. Yet there are dozens of effective treatments that can be used, only the doctor is unaware of them and the patient is also unaware of them as well.

Eastern medicine includes natural herbs, acupuncture, and tai chi in the healing of illness. This involves the concept of restoring balance in the body thus restoring the health of the body. Then there is also the spiritual side of healing and the use of the priesthood in healing people who are sick. But I imagine doctors will not suggest giving priesthood blessings to their patients. In some cases if the doctor is LDS and the patients are LDS this might be the case. My wife's doctor did suggest this before she had surgery. Maybe during the millennium this will be the case, but by that time people may not need medical treatment.

It is wonderful to be able to have readily access to medical emergencies from 911, and being able to treat things that are beyond our control with modern medicine, but there is a better way of living and a better way to health then waiting until we get sick to start to think about our health. We can live better lives and more enjoyable lives by being healthy, and the best part of it is that it doesn't cost anything, and might even save you a lot of money that you would otherwise spend on medicine, or on visits to the doctor.

My Story

There have been several things in my life that have compelled me to become healthier. It hasn't been until later on in my adulthood that I have been able to understand health better, and I still have a lot of things about health I do not understand yet. I am still learning things every year about health and have applied this to my life making my quality of life better than it has been before.

When I was young, I was like most other kids my age, I played and got sick. My parents would give me something from the medicine cabinet. I would see the doctor if it was a little more serious than normal. If I got injured, I just had to take care of it myself, unless it was a deep cut and then I was taken to the doctor to get stitches which happened twice during my childhood. Once when I had a baseball hit me in the mouth and my teeth went into my lips and the dentist stitched me up, the other time was when I was ducking under the telephone cord back when telephones had cords and hit my head on the corner of my mother's china hutch. It split my head open and my mom took me to the doctor's to get stitches on my head.

It seemed like I was always falling down and getting hurt, but I had never broken a bone, or at least I never was treated for a broken bone. I might have had minor fractures that were healed without medical attention. For the most part, I was responsible for my own health and illnesses and did not go to my parents and tell them I was sick and needed to go to the doctor and take medicine. In fact I did not like to go to the doctor, and did not like taking medicines. I would just go around sick waiting to get better. The most common treatment I went through was rest and chicken noodle soup.

But the thing that bugged me the most was just being sick in the first place. I hated to get sick and I would get sick two to three times a year often lasting more than a week. This meant that I was sick at least one month out of the year. It was a miserable month as well. I was beginning to think that this was common, and that everyone got sick like this, and in fact most of the people I knew would get sick like me especially during the late fall and through the winter known as the flu season.

The worst was when I threw up and had dry heaves, I felt like I was dying when this occurred. It was at those times in my life that I really wanted to know why I got sick and what I could do to prevent it, not treat it, but prevent it from ever happening again. I would start to investigate why I was getting sick and what if anything would help me from getting sick again. At the time there was no internet, and very few computers around, and I was not comfortable looking up things in the library, so I did not do a lot of research. The only thing I could do was to ponder my own health and do things through trial and error. I had heard about how exercise was good, and eating a healthy diet was good, so I started with these and started to exercise and eat right. Only I did not know anything about eating right, and I was limited to what my mom served the family for dinner. I have always had a sweet tooth and took the opportunity to eat sweets whenever I could.

When I was growing up candy and sweets were not as readily available either, and expensive, so my parents did not buy a lot of sweets, pop, or ice cream, and they lives by the old school of not allowing their children to have any candy or sweets unless it was a special occasion or they felt like it. I remember hearing the ice cream pale being opened at night when I went to bed by my parents who would have ice cream after us kids went to bed because they did not want us to have some. So I did not have a lot of sweets as a kid, and I started to exercise.

There were other reasons why I would exercise, one was that I was bullied at school and wanted to be tough to that I would not get bullied anymore, also I thought that girls would like me if I was strong. The only problem was that in elementary, I did not really know how to exercise. I hated running so, I did not run, and I remember that I was so slow when I did run that I left early one day to go home because they were testing all of the kids in the presidential fitness run, and I did not want to be embarrassed by the run.

The only thing I did know about exercise was sit-ups, push-ups, and pull-ups. I went about doing these every day, and became good at doing them. This was during the time when all of the Rocky movies came out, so I started to do one arm push-ups to impress the other kids. I became stronger, a little healthier, only I still got sick, and I was also depressed. It was during this time, I continued to do my own research and pondering about health. I got into bodybuilding in junior high again because I wanted to catch the eye of girls.

It was through body building I learned the important of exercising and proper diet, but of which I worked on. I started to run and do endurance exercises. I also found that I was feeling better, and not just physically but mentally as well. By the time I was in ninth grade I was big into exercise to the point that it made me feel tremendously better than I had before, and I was hooked for the rest of my life on exercise. I was not eating as healthy as I should have been, but my exercise was about where I needed it. I found that through exercising I was less sick than I had been before.

I was involved with football which motivated me to continue to exercise to be in shape for football. Even though I was not able to be on the firs string in high school, I was able to have more of a desire to exercise in my life. It helped me in so many different ways like feeling better mentally and being healthier physically. It also helped to control my ADD, which I never knew I had until later on in my life.

So I was compelled to have a better life by exercising and improving my health. Unknown to me at the time, I was also helping to improve my mental and spiritual health as well. Even though it would take me nearly twenty years before I was able to understand how mental and spiritual health works.

My journey into learning about health continued to grow with each year. I got into learning all I could about nutrition, exercise, and ways to be healthier. I also got into martial arts which seemed to have some important things about health that I thought was very cool at the time. Through martial arts I learned about Eastern medicine with herbs and Tai Chi. There were several points in my life where I have been excited about health and could have gone into the health profession only things happened that I cannot explain and I ended up seeking to be a teacher.

Through my journey of health, I was also beginning to notice my family and friends and all of the health related issues they went through. I wanted to help them as well, only when I would make suggestions they would often argue with me or ignore my advice so I stopped trying, but I wanted desperately to share with them some of the things I was learning about health.

After two years of teaching geography, I was hired on at a school to teach health. This gave me an opportunity to learn more about health, and to be able to teach 8th graders about health. I was able to start thinking about health in a holistic manner. I realized that physical, mental, and spiritual health was connected with each other and if one was affected then the rest were also affected.

There have been several things that I have learned about health that I have never heard a doctor, or read in a text book on health talk about. Yet these things are just as important or even more important to overall health than exercise, nutrition, and reducing stress. This is why it is important to have an open mind when it comes to health, to have the necessary resources, and to have different perspectives. When it comes to health there is thousands of years of understanding health at our fingertips in books, on the internet, and in our own mind and body we are able to tap into a vast amount of knowledge. We also have the ability to look at things on a spiritual level which many people dismiss, but more important than eating the right foods, exercise, and getting enough sleep.

Through experience and research, I know our health can be a function of our own will and determination. There are countless stories of survival and endurance that defies current medial knowledge. I have been able to push myself and overcome a lot of health issues in my life that I see other people would not be able to do. If there is a will there is a way to optimum health. You might not be able to be the perfect model, or have the muscles of a bodybuilder or the strength or endurance of an Olympic athlete, but you still can do amazing things with your health if you are willing to give it a try and put forth the effort. Remember there is a price for everything in life. Your health should be one of those things you should be willing to pay the price for. In the end if you do not pay the price of your effort and time, you will be paying for it later in the hospital with money and time that you cannot afford.

It is like having a time machine. If you had a heart attack and knew what you needed to do to prevent it and could go back in time to take the necessary steps to prevent it would you do it. Most of us would go back in time and do what we could to prevent it, knowing that we will have the heart attack if we do nothing. Well we all have that opportunity to change the future or plan our future by our lifestyle now.

One thing that I have struggled with for many years is to see the health of my family and friends deteriorate with age. Sure there is a natural process where the body starts to age and health diminishes, but I have seen it too many times when the people I care about gain a lot of extra weight and start to have many ailments, which I believe could be reversed or made better through exercise, diet, stress management, and spiritual exercise. I am frustrated because I know what it is like to have good health, and it makes me feel sad that I am unable to help my family and friends because they do not have the time or the will power to make the changes necessary in their lifestyles.

I have also found that it is nearly impossible to get through to family and friends. Family and friends tend to listen to the advice of others than to listen to the advice of someone they know. It is a sense that if you know the person, then that person is somewhat less qualified or knows what they are talking about than a stranger they do not know. People are so eager to jump on to a trend or fad than they are to listen to rational reasoning. They are looking for the quick fix, the magic pill, or the wonder workout that will help them lose weight, look great, and be able to transform their health in as little as twenty minutes a day for four weeks. Results will vary. The truth of the matter is the results will be different for everyone.

There is no wonder drug, perfect workout, or fad that will bring about overall health in your life. It takes years of dedication and commitment to be able to have a lifestyle that works for you and will give you optimum health. You might say that this is crazy and there is no way you will invest years in something you do not know will even work. The bottom line is that you are not just investing year, but the rest of your life devoted to improving your overall health, and the beauty of it is that it doesn't really cost anything except for time, and a commitment to be healthier.

All of the things in this book are not new. There is no secret or special diet, exercise routine, or crazy idea that will help you have better health. It is all just common sense and a matter of making your health practices work for you. Some people might be able to eat a certain diet, but others might be allergic to what the person is eating. Some people can ride bikes and run, others can only walk. Part of the process of being healthy is to come up with things that is perfect for you.

You are the one in charge of your health, not your doctor, not the fitness instructor, not me. It is your responsibility as a parent, spouse, friend, and human being to work towards being healthy so that you can play with your children, help those who need help, and live a long healthy productive happy life.

To Do List

1. Practice being aware of all areas of your health.
2. Work on having good posture and sitting correctly, the spine is the central communications link between the brain and the rest of the body. If the spine is injured or not healthy then it affects general health. Many people have back problems because they have poor posture and sit incorrectly.
3. Practice proper breathing through the nose not the mouth. Proper breathing is known as belly or stomach breathing where you allow the breath to be able to raise and lower your stomach. This breathing will allow you to get more oxygen. You will have more energy and less headaches and it will help you to be able to get over an illness much faster.
4. Be mindful of the things you do each day and pay attention to those things that effect your health such as the thoughts that go through your mind, and how you interact with others.
5. Examine your daily routines and see if any of it has to do with health, or if some of it might be modified.
6. Limit the amount of time you spend in front of the television and the amount of time you spend on the computer on the internet. This can free up some time for you to be able to exercise or be able to do other things in your life that will help you to improve your health.
7. Examine your sleep patterns. Do you go to bed the same time and wake up the same time each day? Are you staying up late a lot?

Chapter Two: LDS Perspective on Health

"And all saints who remember to keep and do these
sayings, walking in obedience to the commandments shall
receive health in their navel and marrow to their bones;
And shall find wisdom and great treasures of knowledge,
even hidden treasures; And shall run and not be weary, and
shall walk and not faint." (D&C 89:18-20)

When members of the church think of the church's
view of health the first thing that comes to mind is the
Word of Wisdom which outlines a lot of things in regards
to health mainly focusing on diet and what not to consume.
But it is so much more than just diet, and just the Word of
Wisdom that brings in the LDS perspective on health.
Many other religions have health guidelines like the Jewish
law of having food prepared in a certain way and restricting
the consumption of certain foods like pork. Islam also has a
similar law that is like the Jewish law, and they also forbid
the consumption of alcohol.

When we look at health in the church we can see
that members of the church who follow the Word of
Wisdom tend to be healthier than those who do not. But
again there is more to health in the church than just the
Word of Wisdom and being forbidden to use harmful
substances in our body. There are many of the practices in
the church that promote health.

With the youth of the church there is the, "For the
Strength of Youth," pamphlet for the youth of the church to
read and follow. It is a great resource for parents and their
children to be able to have access to what the church says
about spiritual, social, mental, and physical health. It gives
a good overall path or direction youth can take to be
healthy.

In the young men's program boys go through scouts
which encourages good health through proper diet, better

living, and outdoor recreation like camping and hiking. The church also includes sports in the young men's program which helps them to get more exercise and be excited about exercising. Many of the young men are involved in other sports and activities as well. In the Duty to God program young men starting at age 12 are required to do things to improve spiritual health as well as physical health.

I have personally been involved with scouting, and the young men's program and there are a lot of things that I have taught the young men of the church about overall health. It is a good program to help young men learn about how to take care of themselves, and those that are not able to go through scouts, or get their Duty to God are missing out on a lot of knowledge, skills, and help to get them on the right path to health for a lifetime.

In the young women's program they are also encouraged to be healthy and make healthy decisions in their life. They also play sports and are encouraged to live a healthy life. The Personal Progress program for young women to receive their Young Women's Medallion goes through several virtues they are suppose to pass off which involved a lot of service and spiritual habits that helps the young women in social and spiritual health.

I am not surprised that the youth of the church are among the healthiest in the world with the training and habits they receive while they are young. Even when the youth reach missionary age they are encouraged to be healthy so that they are able to serve a mission without health problems. Then when they serve a mission they have to keep themselves healthy by following a strict routine of getting up early, eating healthy, and walking or biking around their area to meet with people and teach the gospel to others.

As adults in the church there are also a lot of things that are emphasized that relate to overall health. Each stake has adult sports programs, and many wards do activities that involve social interaction which helps people to connect with each other and share idea. For many people in the church, the church is a key social health center than encourages interaction and service to others. A member of the church cannot be a member of the church without having a calling. Every man in the church is a home teacher, and every woman a visiting teacher. Just in these callings it encourages social interaction with families and members of the church. It can also include compassionate service and help those in need.

When it comes to health there are some definite targeted area the church focuses on with the Word of Wisdom and diet, there is the emphasis on exercise, education, compassionate service, and many other things the church does including emergency training and preparedness. So when it comes to health, the LDS perspective is universal and holistic health that gives its members an advantage over non-members.

But just like in everything in life, Satan and his followers are busy tempting and attacking church members in the area of health. If Satan can get a member to break the Word of Wisdom or to have them start to do an unhealthy habit then he has won the battle and claimed another victim. To follow the gospel's teachings is to be healthy and do what we can to remain that way, unfortunately being healthy takes work and effort, which makes it difficult for many people to put forth the effort to be healthy.

The world is becoming a very unhealthy place to live in. There are many different aspects of the world that are very unhealthy, only there is a false sense of security with all of the emphasis on nutrition and exercise we might see in the media and at school. The social and moral fabric of society is destroying families and people's spiritual health.

Just taking a look at the energy drinks that are being sold, many members of the church may think that it is okay to drink them, especially since they are promoted as being healthy, and gives you energy. There is a media blitz saying green tea is really healthy for you. Yet, those energy drinks contain high amounts of sugar and caffeine and have been proven to be unhealthy. We have been encouraged by prophets to not take anything into our bodies that is harmful to them. Tea and coffee has been identified by church leaders as being on the list of harmful substances. We can also argue that eating chocolate cake and ice cream is bad for you. The idea in many cases is to examine your lifestyle and look at those habits that might be unhealthy and then start to change them. It might not be a commandment to not to drink an energy drink, but it is a commandment to treat your body as a temple, and taking something that can harm your body can be considered a sin.

The intent is a big part of it as well. When you do something what is your intent. Is your intend selfish to indulge in self gratification without any regard for your health and others, or is your intend just to celebrate someone's birthday with a little ice cream and cake. There is also the idea of being able to live without something and determining if you are addicted to something. If it is really hard for you to give up something then you might be addicted to it, and it can be harmful to your health.

Church Members

As church members we might look at health in terms of what not to take or do that might harm our health. If a member was asked what to do to be healthy they would say something like eat right, exercise, and then talk about not drinking alcohol, smoking, and doing drugs. A young child would repeat what they have learned in primary class about the Word of Wisdom.

I smiled when I overheard my daughter at age six talking to her friend about how smoking was bad for people and that people should not smoke because it was not good for their health. I am not sure if she and her friend understood why smoking was not good or even fully understood the Word of Wisdom, but at least something sunk in. They also talked about how saying bad words was not good either. They did not associate it with health, but they knew that saying bad words was not good. I am not sure even adults know that the words we say or hear affects our health as well. A great deal of our mental health and spiritual health is affected by the words we hear and say.

Think about the damage verbal abuse has had on children and adults. It is huge when it comes to mental health as well as spiritual health, yet many people will not mention words as being part of health. We teach how we should speak and act from our lessons in church and from our scripture study and listen modern day prophets talk about these things, but I am not sure if we know its impact on our health.

There are a lot of things in the church that as members we are taught that relates to our health, but do not associate it with health. This is something that we need to be aware of and not just accept it as something that was said in church or during conference. It gives more depth to what is being taught in the gospel.

Originally the Word of Wisdom was taught as something the members of the church should start to follow. Many of the members did not fully embrace it or believe that it had much to do with their salvation and health. There had not been any studies or research on the affects of alcohol and tobacco back in the 1800's. Many of the people had seen the effects of alcohol and new that it was not good for someone to get drunk, and they knew how disgusting tobacco could be. Emma complained to Joseph about having to clean up after the mess the brethren made during their meetings. Yet the Word of Wisdom was not yet fully realized.

Today we see the full impact of the Word of Wisdom and have gained the great treasures of knowledge spoken of in the passage. I am certain there are many more of the scripture that will be revealed and the modern day prophets have said much more about it. It has become a catalyst or springboard for healthy practices in the church.

Yet when we look at health as members of the church, everything in the church affects health in one way or another. It might be spiritual health we are working on, mental health, physical health, social health, or even financial health. All of these things are important and when one suffers they all suffer. It is one thing that as members of the church we need to recognize and understand so that we are in the process of working on overall health in our lives and understand that if we are depressed it will affect our spiritual as well as our physical health too.

The church sets the standard when it comes to health and the world has to slowly catch up. The Lord knows what is best for us and the best way for us to have ultimate health. He is all knowing when it comes to everything in the Universe including health, and so it makes sense to follow his plan when it comes to health and not to look to fad diets or people who are just wanting to make money off of your desire to be thin, look good, or have a healthy life.

The Ways of the World

As members of the church, we can look at what the world thinks of health with an LDS perspective that comes from the Lord. We do not have to be health fanatics to be healthy, in fact many of the leaders of the church have spoken against being fanatical about health. So when there is a trend for people to become vegetarians it talks about in the Doctrine and Covenants about that it is wrong to become a vegetarian and it is okay to eat meat.

When a new fad comes out all we have to do is look to the modern prophets for advice. There are many times in general conference where they will address such issues that comes up like with piercings and tattoos. We as members can also access personal revelation and ask when we are not sure about a product we might have a question about or a certain practice. It is a mistake to take the word of others about things. Fast and pray for the answers to your questions. It might be that something might be okay for someone when it comes to health and not okay for another person. Just like how rock climbing is a great form of exercise and recreation, but it is not for everyone.

When it comes to health, it really is a personal matter and personal preferences. It doesn't meant that you get to indulge in unhealthy practices, but it does mean that you need to develop your own exercise routine, and some of the other healthy routines in your life. This is something more and more people are starting to do, only the ways of the world are not the ways of the church, and it is important to understand this.

The world might be following energy drinks and green tea as the new healthy thing to do. But it is just like the studies of wine and alcohol that say it is healthy for you to drink small amounts of. Just because they do a study that has some correlation between drinking some wine for dinner and a healthy heart does not mean that it is okay to drink alcohol and break the word of wisdom because some researcher says it is okay. We have access to modern day scriptures, prophets and personal revelation. The ways of the world doesn't have this.

We do not have to argue what is healthy and not healthy, we just have to follow the ways of the church and be obedient to the commandments of the Lord including the words of the modern day prophets. Everything in the church affects our spiritual health which in turns affects our physical and overall health. So when it comes to health we just need to be guided by the doctrines of the church.

Then why is it so hard to be healthy these days. Part of the reason why we are here on the earth is to receive physical bodies, and the other part is to prepare to meet God, both of which has to do with health and healthy living. Satan on the other hand wants to destroy our spiritual health and will do it in any means he can including destroying our physical health as well.

I heard a member of the church tell me and my companion on my mission that she could not understand how a loving Heavenly Father would hold smoking against someone when it came to entering into the Kingdom of God. She talked about how she couldn't understand how it would be part of the judgment. In her mind she couldn't believe that someone would be condemned because they smoked. She then talked about how there are a lot of really bad people in the world who cheat, lie, steal, and hurt other people, but to condemn someone just because they have a bad habit was not something she was willing to accept.

At the time we really did not have any real answers to her questions, except that it is a commandment and people who smoke are being disobedient to the commandment. But we did not change her mind when it came to her belief that smoking was a spiritual issue. We could have gone further to explain how our bodies are temples and we should not hurt them, but I doubt that she would have accepted that line of reasoning either.

The question is if we are doing things that make us unhealthy are we committing a sin and will it affect our salvation? I would not be the first one to jump at the chance to judge anyone when it came to health issues. But I do judge myself and look at my life and my health to see if I am doing the right things. There are many times when I find myself indulging in too much ice cream or being a little too lazy, but when I do these things is it sin? Am I disobeying a commandment and breaking the Word of Wisdom? There have been times when I have gone into a temple recommend interview with a glimmer of doubt weather I have been living the Word of Wisdom or not.

I believe that in many ways some of the things I have done do go against the will of the Lord and I have in a way broken the Word of Wisdom when it comes to the idea of trying to be healthy and not harm my body which was given to me by my Father in Heaven and is considered a temple. I feel that I need not confess these things to my bishop, but that these things are between me and the Lord. When I am talking some of the things I have done, they are not terrible sins that would warrant a confession to a priesthood leader, but minor infractions that have diminished not only my physical health, but my spiritual health as well.

It is the difference between someone who strictly observes the Sabbath day by not going shopping, going out to play basketball, and spends the day attending meetings, holding family council, going home teaching or visiting teaching, and reading the scriptures, praying, and fasting, and someone who attends church, but then spends the rest of the time in front of the television watching football, or goes out to eat at a restaurant.

We will all be judged according to our intent. A person will not be condemned for eating a little too much ice cream, but for that moment of indulgence the person might not be able to listen to the spirit as well as a person who is not overeating. Despite the degree of the sins we commit they all affect our spirituality to some extent, and if we continue to live a lifestyle that is not in harmony with the spirit, then we will not have those blessings in our life.

Living a healthy lifestyle for a member of the church, does not just mean abstaining from harmful substances, it means living healthy so that as members of the church we can have access to the great knowledge spoken of in the Word of Wisdom. It means that when we have retired we are healthy enough to serve a mission with our spouse. It means that we will be healthy enough to be around for our grandchildren and be able to help teach them the gospel. As members of the church we are among the healthiest people of the world, but that doesn't mean it doesn't take effort to get there.

Many members of the church fall into the same traps people around the world fall into when it comes to health especially in the United States where there is over 30 percent obesity among adults and 17 percent for children. Health is not just an ideal that we sometimes think might be unattainable it is a way of life, and a commandment of the Lord. Part of our learning process on this earth is to understand our bodies, understand our spirits, and minds. It is a time to prepare to meet God, not in a sad and fallen state, but a joyous healthy state where we have not only learned the ways of the Lord in spiritual ways, but also in all aspects of our health.

As Latter-day Saints we need to understand that health includes all aspects of our lives both spiritual and physical. Without one the other is injured. We must not only practice those things in our lives that our spiritual, but we also need to work on our physical and mental health as well. It is important to read scriptures on a daily basis, but it is also important to be active and eat healthy on a daily basis as well. If we were to make this part of our lives then we will not only be healthier we will have greater access to happiness and the Holy Ghost in our lives. We will receive a lot more blessings that will enable us to do things we never thought possible.

Those hidden treasures spoken of in the Word of Wisdom are things that only you can find out by living the Word of Wisdom. With health as well as personal revelation you have access to something only the Lord will reveal to you. It might be that you will discover a talent you never knew you had, or a new direction your life is going to take. It may simply unlocking the mysteries of health for you and being able to overcome a chronic illness, get energy you never thought possible. Be able to live life free of pain and illness.

Some would believe that heaven is only a place where you go to after you have died if you are worth to go there. Others believe you can create your own heaven while still on earth. People can certainly create their own hell on earth why not heaven. A student I had in school made a comment that he believed that we created our own destiny after we die, that what we have here on earth was what we had when we died. This I believe is true. There are certain elements that will be different like the absence of temptation, and we will all have immortal bodies. But our bodies and our life after we die will be in part to what we have done while we were on this earth, and it will mark our progression on the other side. When we die it is not the end of life, but a beginning.

It will be the beginning of our eternal lives which is infinite. What we have learned and have done in this life will be where we start in the next, which means that those who did not do a lot in this life and did not learn many of the important lessons will need to learn then in the next life. Everyone will be in a different point in their eternal progression, even in families each will be at a different spot. Those who have inherited the celestial kingdom will have a different level or progression within the kingdom which will be endless. Those who have inherited lesser kingdoms will not have the opportunity to progress beyond their kingdoms, and in many causes it might be that their will and what they have done on this earth confines them to a state of damnation.

I have seen this among the students I have taught, where some do not care about school, and think it is a joke.

They sit around and do nothing and complain about how boring the class is. I tell them that if they did any work then they would not be so bored. I also ask then what they do at home or during the summer and their response is that they do nothing. Later I run into these students and find out that they haven't done much with their lives. I can imagine that they would be perfectly content sitting around through eternity not doing anything while others are progressing and learning the wisdom of the heavens. To me not doing anything for eternity would be hell.

While on my mission, me and my companion were teaching a Muslim man about the gospel and we asked him what he thought the afterlife was like. He described what he called a paradise where he would be free to do everything he did while he was on the earth without any restrictions and without any pain, suffering, illness, and conflict with others. He described a place that was his heaven, which I believe will be his heaven if he were to continue to live the way he did.

In other words what we do in this life will affect the next. It might be that we have to overcome an unhealthy habit in the next life in order to move on with our progression. It might be that we have to learn lessons on how to have a better relationship with others, or be more obedient to the commandments of the Lord. Some might then have a perspective that it is okay to do what we want in this life, because we would have eternity to fix our mistakes. This kind of thinking is folly, because our intent and actions in this life sets the stage for the next.

It is like those students in my classroom who do not do their work and fail my class. They believe they will be able to make it up later, and be able to get their GED or something as an equivalent, but what happens to them is that they go through the horrors of trying to find a job, having to struggle financially for years, going from one relationship to the next and never knowing true love. Even if they finally intend on getting more education and turning their life around it is far harder to them then if they were to just have done the work in my class in the first place.

It is far better if you live this life well by following the commandments of the Lord, than if you attempt to follow them later in eternity. Even people who have committed sins early in life and attempt to repent of them later suffer tremendously to get back to the gospel. It is difficult for them to return to the church and resume their life. It is important to continue to follow the teaching of the modern prophets now and receive the blessings then to miss out on the blessings and suffer the pains of hell.

Part of this journey through life and following the modern day prophets and the commandments of the Lord is to have a healthy lifestyle. Throughout the history of the world the Lord has given prophetic council to his saints to be healthy in terms of spiritual, physical, and mental health. We often overlook the subtle scriptural passages of health, and forget that many of the prophets followed a healthy lifestyle. There are many passages in the scriptures that we will explore in order to come to a more full understanding of the relationship with the gospel and our health.

It is the LDS perspective of health that makes the difference when it comes to health. The world will continue to go through its fad diets, periods of excess and periods of fanaticism that mark how people look at health. There are many things of health that have always been part of living healthy and predate scientific studies thousands of years. It is our responsibility to unlock the mysteries of heaven in relation to our own health.

Satan has used health and the misuse of it to destroy people's lives and drag many people down through the depths of hell. There is nothing faster than to drag a faithful member of the church down in the depths of sin than to get him addicted to alcohol, tobacco, or other illegal substances. A person who is breaking the Word of Wisdom is selfish only thinking of their own desire to have another drink, smoke another cigarette, and take more of the addictive substance without any regard to their own health and how it is affecting the other people in their lives. Satan does not want us to be happy, and by destroying our health he can do this.

Have you ever seen a drug addict who was truly happy? Getting pleasure from a drug is not happiness. Those who are unhealthy tend to be unhealthy in many other ways through the abuse of family and friends. Often you can recognize someone who is not living a healthy life by the how happy they are and how their spirituality is.

I have seen people at the store who are dirty, a lot of missing teeth, and everything about them is telling me that they are not health physically, spiritually, or mentally. If I were to follow these people, I would hear a vocabulary that is very demeaning for them and those around them. They are constantly verbally abusing those around them without even knowing it, and they are also abusing their children through second hand smoke or through neglect by buying alcoholic beverages instead of food for dinner. These people are so addicted to their lifestyle that they fail to recognize what they are doing to the people around them, and fail to recognize themselves in the mirror. If they were to just start by living a healthier lifestyle they would start changing the way they think, speak, and act around others.

Each year when I start to get to know my students, I can pick out the students who are members of the church or who have a healthier lifestyle just by seeing how they dress, their actions in class, and how they treat others. There is even a level of appearance among the 11 year old scouts that I have taught. Those who are healthier seem to shine more than those who are not. They are at a higher level than those who do not take care of themselves.

When it comes to being healthy, those who are healthy are happier, more positive, willing to help others, willing to work hard, are more knowledgeable, and are more spiritual than those who are not as healthy. There are some exceptions to this, like those who are born with a chronic illness, or those who have been living a healthy lifestyle and suddenly get cancer, or get into an accident. This is a natural part of human existence where we struggle with health issues. I have found that it is how we face these challenges that matters. Those who are born with health issues have often been given a spiritual shield that enables them to go throughout life without being affected by the temptations of Satan.

Sometimes people are given physical illnesses to become humble and to seek out the Lords help in order to overcome the illness. So illness comes to each of us to help teach us about life and about the ways in which the Lord's plan works in our lives. I have seen people with cancer, and people who are about to die healthier than those who do not have cancer and are not about to die, because they are spiritually healthier than other people. A person who abuse their bodies, minds, and spirit look far unhealthier than those who work to be healthy, do everything in their power to help their family, and live a spiritual life than those who don't.

It then becomes a question of defining health. Is health being free from illness and living a long life, or is it being happy and doing the things you want to do. I watched as my grandparents from my mother's side go through a lot of health issues, yet they were always happy and spent a lot of time with family and going on vacations. They enjoyed life, even though my grandfather went through a lot of health issues when it came to his heart and eventually dies of heart disease. My grandmother also went through a lot of health issues and eventually died from cancer. I know that if they would have eaten better and exercises more they would have been able to live longer and would have had a bigger impact on their grandchildren. They were living healthy spiritual lives, and did their part with family, only they were not living physically healthy lives which had an impact on how long they lived.

My grandmother on my father's side died early on and I never really got to know here. She died from a sudden illness, that she had no control over, but my sisters said that she was always happy and doing crazy things with them. I believe that my father was able to get some of her spirit in him which made it possible for him to be active in the church. Whereas my grandfather was not a member of the church, and did not do much in relation with the church, and I always remembered him sitting around in his house watching television smoking his cigar when we can for a visit. He ended up living to be 90 years old much older than my other grandparents, yet there was something always missing in his life. He never seemed to be happy, and he was not as interactive with grandchildren as my other grandparents. Even though he lived longer, he did not seem healthier than my other grandparents.

I would have to say that a good determination of health has to be happiness and quality of life. If you are happy and the quality of your life is such that you are able to do the things you want to do then you are healthy. Part of life will be to struggle with health related issues, but the more you learn and practice healthy living the more you will be able to gain a greater understanding of the plan of salvation.

Taking an LDS perspective on health we will look at spiritual health and how it relates to overall health. We will look at mental, physical, financial, and social health as well as regards to how the church sees these things. It will give you a better understanding how health and the church are interrelated and how by being healthy you will be able to have greater access to spiritual blessings and personal revelation.

Free Will

We all have free will, or the power to choose. Part of our preparation on this earth is the use of our free will and to be able to make informed decisions about our health as well as spiritual matters. Satan uses our free will to his advantage especially when it comes to our choice of healthy practices. We have the choice between eating healthy foods, or unhealthy ones. We have the choice to exercise each day or to sit around watching television. We have the choice to take a drug or not to take it.

Our lives are filled with difficult choices, and many of them have to do with our health. Just think of all of the choices you have made over the years that have involved family, friends, the church, your diet, your physical activity, and your education all of which is part of your overall health. Satan attempts to persuade you to make the wrong choices in your life by promising pleasures, and enjoyment which is only temporary. The happiness he promises is only temporary and will not last long, and often deepens pain and sorrow that comes from the reality of having poor health.

We have the power within each of us to make the right choices in life, and to be able to live a healthy life and receive all of the blessings that comes from living a healthy life. We are in control of our life and our destiny what happens to us is a result of what we do and the choices we make. Even in situations where people were forced into concentration camps or prisoner of war camps and their health conditions became poor, they had the choice whether to give up and die or have hope and live on until they were rescued. Many of the Jews in World War II and the prisoners of war were able to survive simply because they chose to survive and be able to tell others what went on in those camps. Despite being starved and living in the most horrid of conditions many were able to survive and be able to live long productive lives.

We all die. It doesn't matter how we die, but it matters how we lived and how we spent our years of probation here on earth, preparing to meet God. If we wasted our probation and neglected to do our part and learn as much as we can then we lived and died in vain. But if we took advantage of life and lived life to its fullest, then we have lived a worthwhile life. If we can resist temptation and not allow ourselves to be sucked into the current trends in health, we will be able to live a quality life with the richness of the gospel.

Christ Like Life

In order to be healthy we need to live as the Savior did. He did not have some of the temptations we have life like fast food restaurants, illegal drugs, and a social media that emulates poor behavior. But he did live among a lot of people who had corrupt thoughts and sought to get gain and power over other people. He went through the temptations of food, of living an idol life, and many of the other pitfalls of life in regards to health. In the Garden of Gethsemane he felt all of the sorrows and sins of the world in regards to health, and he knows what each of us go through when we make the wrong decision about our health.

Jesus knew what it was to work hard as a carpenter's son. He knew the traditions of the Jewish diet and the spiritual laws of the time. He went into the wilderness to prepare for his mission by fasting and praying, and was tempted by Satan offering him food, power, and the desires of his heart. Christ was able to rebuke Satan and follow his mission overcoming the cravings of the body and worldly pleasures. He denied himself of food, and the pleasures of the world in order to get closer to his Heavenly Father and to be able to fulfill his mission.

Are you prepared for your mission in life, or are you unable to fulfill your mission, because you are unhealthy to do so? Each of us is given a purpose or mission in life, and if we are unable to fulfill our mission in life then we lose all of the opportunities and blessings in life, and we affect all of the people in our lives as well. It would be a shame if a young man was unable to go on a mission because he was unhealthy. There are situations where things are beyond a person's control when it comes to health, but most of us have control over healthy practices.

The amount of church work we do is a reflection of how healthy we are. We can do a lot of things to help improve our health and thus improve the amount of work we can do in the church and for our families. The Savior when he started his mission was able to serve many people and traveled extensively throughout the region spreading the gospel. John the Baptist was also able to do a lot of preaching of the gospel to help prepare the way for the Lord and lived a healthy life in the wilderness.

Evil Men

"Behold, verily, thus saith the Lord unto you: In the consequence of evils and designs which do and will exist in the hearts of conspiring men in the last days. I have warned you, and forewarn you, by giving you this word of wisdom by revelation." (D&C 89:4)

There are a lot of evil men in the last days who are conspiring to destroy the health of people in order to get wealthy. Many of the money makers are part of selling drugs, or addictive substances including foods that have high amounts of caffeine and sugar. Many people in society especially the poor are addicted to these substances which companies produce for the masses in order to become wealthy and those companies do not care about if their product is healthy or not, in many cases they know that their products are unhealthy and know how it affects the health of others and they still produce their products.

The tobacco company knew that tobacco was harmful to health, and they lied to congress when they said that nicotine was not addictive. There was proof that tobacco companies were targeting children because they were more susceptible and easily persuaded to take something out of rebellion to harm their bodies. One tobacco company even sent a letter to someone in another country encouraging the sale of tobacco products in their country so that it would control the population because it would kill off people. Cigarette smoking has killed more people than Hitler ever did, the only difference is that the owners of the tobacco companies killed people to make money, Hitler had Jewish people killed because he didn't like them.

So when it comes to evil men and women they do not come any more evil than those working for the tobacco companies, the alcohol companies, the pharmaceutical companies, and the food industry where the people are making a profit from the vulnerabilities of people's weaknesses. This is why the Lord gave Joseph Smith the revelation on the Word of Wisdom. To help warm the saints of what these people would be doing in the food industry.

I was appalled by how people go to any lengths to get a fix or high even using such things as bath salts, a combination of herbs called "Spice," and sniffing glue. It seems like every day there is something new that people have come up with that is used from household cleaners, or over the counter medicines to create a toxic substance that alters the mind. It would be easier and less expensive if these people would just run into a brick wall they would have the same results only they would not be as likely to become addicted to running into a brick wall and they would be able to learn from the experience.

There was a story in the news of a girl who had died of an overdose when the couple she was babysitting for gave her drugs. As a parent and a teacher I believe that these people are giving drugs to children are pure evil with their only regard to profit from the weakness of others, and there is a very high price to pay for it as well with the children becoming addicted and ruining their lives. It is sad to hear all of the stories of children who have destroyed their future because of drugs.

Some of the legal products on the shelves are just as addictive with their caffeine and sugar content. I am shocked to hear people who drink a six pack of soda pop every day. I can just imagine how that will affect their health. It might not have any short term side effects, but long term would result in weight gain, diabetes, heart disease, cancer, and a whole host of other illnesses as a result form drinking too much pop.

This is why it is important to teach our children to be healthy and to make the right decisions in their lives regarding their health. Parents need to lead by example, and as members of the church it is our responsibility to be watchful in the things we are buying at the grocery store. I went to the grocery store and bought a cereal, I thought was healthy, only to read the label when I got home to find out that it had green tea in it. I should have taken the cereal back to the grocery store, but I ended up throwing it away. I have seen countless drinks that have tea and caffeine in them and they are promoted as healthy drinks and the label is designed to make you think that it is healthy.

We all know of the alcohol commercial where the people are having fun, and in the movies where people go to a party and they portray drinking as having fun. I fortunately have never had such fun, but have heard and seen how people throw up, act silly, and are in an atmosphere void of the spirit. I cannot imagine having fun making myself sick, and being around other people who are sick, or not acting themselves. Getting into a car accident and killing innocent people is not having fun, and becoming an alcoholic where you sacrifice your family, friends, job, and life to get another drink is not fun either.

There was one homeless man who went into a car station and was given over a thousand dollars by the cashier because she thought he was robbing her. By the time they caught up with the man which was in less than 24 hours he had spent it all on alcohol. So when it comes to evil, destroying a person's health is pure evil. It is easier today to be able to bring someone down through taking things that is harmful to our bodies than it is trying to get someone to rob, lie, cheat, commit adultery, and murder.

In the book *A Long Way Gone: Memoirs of a Boy Soldier*, the author tells how he was recruited into the military and how the military gave them marijuana and cocaine which made them crazy killers. He did a lot of terrible things that he would not have normally done without the drugs. The drug cartels of Mexico and Latin America have not just killed thousands of people in a drug war, they have killed many more and destroyed thousands of lives from the drugs that they sell on the streets. I am horrified by people who claim that it would be better if we were to legalize these drugs in order to put the cartels out of business.

People talk about the failure of prohibition in the United States because of the glorified gangster activities such as Al Capone and his activities in smuggling alcohol. The data at the time did show that drinking had dropped and that prohibition was actually working, only the killings among the mobsters overshadowed the success of the law. I am convinced that the violence of the mobs would have been there with or without prohibition, and it was not the repeal of the law that stopped the violence it was Al Capone being put in jail and the United States declaring war against Japan and Germany that united the country and the mobs went underground for a while.

Gangs and mobs will use anything they can to make money and exploit people no matter what laws are made. It takes the diligence of the community to get rid of them that makes the difference. This is why the church is so important when it comes to health and healthy living. The church is not only a means to warm the members of unhealthy practices, it is a way for people to fight against the evil people of the world who would come to destroy them.

To Do List

1. Examine the different things in your life that relates to the gospel and how many of them relate to your overall health.
2. Take a look at those things that are in the media or in your community that come from the evil designs of men in order to hurt your health.
3. Reexamine your health in terms of the gospel and look at Spiritual things first before thinking about them in terms of physical health.
4. Read section 89 in the Doctrine and Covenants again in terms of the Word of Wisdom and study its contents.
5. Explore the scriptures in terms of your health to see what the Lord says about the different areas of health
6. Study what modern day prophets tell us about health in past issues of the Ensign with conference talks these can be accessed on the Church's website.
7. When looking at health always keep in mind the gospel first. Seek the Kingdom of God and all other things will be added to you.

Chapter Three: Spiritual Health

"For by the power of my Spirit created I them; yea,
all things both spiritual and temporal-First spiritual,
secondly temporal, which is the beginning of my work…"
(D&C 29:31-32)

Everything was first created spiritually and then temporally or physically. Thus when we start to look at health we need to first look at spiritual health. It is spiritual health that sets the foundation of all other health and takes precedence. For many members of the church being spiritually healthy simply means reading scriptures daily, having regular prayer, magnifying their callings, and doing church service. But there are a lot more things that involve spiritual health, and a lot of ways spiritual health will impact the other parts of your health as well.

People who are not following the gospel will become depressed because they are not following their true self, and then with depression they get physically ill being exhausted and sick most of the time. It will also affect their social health as well, because people do not like to be around depressed people, and depressed people do not like to be around other people, especially people who seem happy because it reminds them of something they believe they cannot have.

You can often see people who are not spiritually healthy, because it affects the rest of their health. It doesn't matter what the person's status is in life, where they are from, or what ethnic group they are. A person who is spiritually unhealthy will not be happy, blame others for their misfortunes, be envious of others who have more than they do, will be upset mentally, will not take care of their physical health often being dirty, using alcohol, tobacco, and caffeine in their lives in order to numb their existence.

They will be fearful of the light and anything to do with kindness, and wholesome living. The people will latch on to people who are just as spiritually dead as they are, who speak as they do, and have the same filthy habits as they do. They mock those who have more spiritual light than they do and refuse to take any part of the gospel. It is not until they humble themselves and seek out the light that they are able to start to change.

So with spiritual health the foundation and with it affecting so many other things, let's start with looking at spiritual health and to see how to strengthen it and make our spiritual health stronger in our lives. All things start with spirituality.

Who are you?

"The Spirit itself beareth witness with our spirit, that we are the children of God: And if children, then heirs; heirs of God, and joint-heirs with Christ; if so be that we suffer with him, that we may be also glorified together." (Romans 8:16-17)

We are spirit children of our Heavenly Father and heirs to what he has. Just like our earthly father we can become like him and have all that he has. In the preexistence before we can to the earth we existed as a spirit son and daughter to our Father in Heaven. We were also given a mission to fulfill while we were here on this earth.

"Before I formed thee in the belly I knew thee; and before thou camest forth out of the womb I sanctified thee and I ordained thee…" (Jeremiah 1:5)

In the preexistence we learned and grew as spirit children, but we did not have bodies and so our progression was not complete we still needed a body in order to learn and to grow and to be like our Father and Heaven who has a glorified body. Therefore following the plan that was accepted by us, we came to this earth and received a mortal body. This was because of our first parents in the garden of Eden Adam and Eve who partook of the fruit of the Tree of the knowledge of Good and Evil which caused them to become mortal and subject to physical death and a separation of them from the presence of Heavenly Father causing a spiritual death for them because of their disobedience, thus requiring repentance and a Savior in order to save us from our sins.

We are then spiritual beings having a physical experience on earth. Our spirits have inherited these bodies, and when we die they will leave the bodies to rot in the earth and be reunited with their bodies during the resurrection in a glorified resurrected state. At that time we will not have to worry so much about physical health because we will then become immortal. This is why it is important that we first look at our spirits and strive to keep our spirits healthy. It is important that we follow Him and his commandments.

"According as he hath chosen us in him before the foundation of the world, that we should be holy and without blame before him in love:" (Ephesians 1:4)

As spiritual beings we have the potential to become like our spiritual Father who is in heaven. This means that we have a lot of potential and will be able to do a lot of great things including being healthy. There are many possibilities when it comes to our spirits. We can do a lot of great things. But it is important to be able to follow God's plan for us in order for us to reap what we sow and receive spiritual blessings.

It is important to be able to do all that we can to let our light shine and help others on the road as well. It is not enough to sit back idly knowing what we know and not to share it with others. This is why missionary work is so vital to not only helping others learn about the gospel, but for our own salvation as well, and to help our personal health.

"Let your light so shine before men, that they may see your good works, and glorify your Father which is in heaven." (Matthew 5:16)

As you let your light shine with your good works, you will grow closer to your Heavenly Father and be able to receive the blessings from heaven to bless your life and your health. The more you let your light shine the more you will be bathed in the light and the healthier your spirit will be. It does take a lot of hard work to get there and to be able to then share your good works with others.

President Monson is the perfect example of this. His light shined bright before he became president of the church. Back when he was a bishop of his ward he let his light shine as he visited all of the widows in his ward and served the Lord as a faithful bishop. His entire life has been filled with service and compassion to others. It isn't any wonder that he has lived a long healthy life and the Lord has supported and blessed him with good health so that he can continue to bless others.

We must get to know our spirits, because they ultimately are interconnected with our physical bodies. "For man is spirit. The elements are eternal, and the spirit and element, inseparably connected, receive a fullness of joy." (D&C 93:33)

The body cannot exist without the spirit and the spirit cannot have a fullness of joy without the body. Christ himself have to take upon himself a body of flesh in order to fulfill all righteousness. He would not have been able to have been baptized of John, have suffered the pains of hunger in the wilderness, walked among the people of his land preaching the gospel, called his twelve apostles, or paid for the sins of the world in the Garden of Gethsemane. But without his spirit he would not have been able to do any of what he had done.

Holy Ghost

"But the fruit of the spirit is love, joy, peace, longsuffering, gentleness, goodness, faith, meekness, temperance; against there is no law." (Galatians 5:22-23)

The Holy Ghost is the essence of the qualities listed above. If those qualities are present then the Holy Ghost is there. A healthy spirit will exhibit those qualities. People who are filled with love, joy, peace, longsuffering, gentleness, goodness, faith, meekness, and temperance are spiritually healthy. Thos who do not possess these qualities are not spiritually healthy and do not have the Holy Ghost with them. It is when the Holy Ghost or the Light of Christ is withdrawn from a person that they are not spiritually healthy.

It is through the Holy Ghost that we receive our strength and power to be healthy, to have personal revelation to guide and direct our lives in such a way that we are healthy. After baptism we are given the baptism of fire which is the Holy Ghost. We are given a direct link to our Father and Heaven and Jesus Christ through the Holy Ghost who guides and directs each of us in the way we should go.

The Holy Ghost fulfills so many roles in our lives. He is the comforter who comes to us when we need comfort from the grief of losing loved ones, or go through chronic illness that causes us a lot of pain. He is the source of our testimonies providing us with the revelation that confirms our faith in the gospel. We receive our spiritual gifts through the Holy Ghost which helps us to fulfill our mission on the earth.

Spiritual Law

"Wherefore, verily I say unto you that all thins unto me are spiritual, and not at any time have I given unto you a law which was temporal…" (D&C 29:34)

Spiritual law governs the universe including all other aspects of health. This means that if spiritual laws are followed then it will bring blessings of better health if spiritual laws are broken those blessings of health will be taken away. It is then important to flow the spiritual laws through obedience to those laws. This is why obedience is spoken of throughout the scriptures. Without being obedient to the commandments of the Lord you will lose your spirituality.

It is through our obedience to these laws that we strengthen our spirits and make them healthier. Just the simple act of obedience allows us to develop spiritual habits that will help to make our spirits healthier. Like with other healthy practices of exercise and eating right it is important to develop a habit of obedience to the commandments and ordinances of the gospel. Without obedience our spirits would withdraw from the Lord and our spirits would grow weak and our health would suffer.

"There is a law, irrevocably decreed in heaven before the foundations of this world, upon which all blessings are predicated." (D&C 130:20)

All blessings including blessings of good health come from this law. Therefore by following the laws of the gospel we can expect to have good health. "For all who have a blessing at my hands shall abide the law which was appointed for that blessing, and the conditions thereof, as were instituted from before the foundation of the world." (D&C 132:5) If you want that blessing you have to obey the law the blessing is associated with.

Since all of the laws of heaven are interconnected it is important to obey all of the laws or commandments of the gospel. If you only choose to obey the law of the fast and pay fast offerings and tithing you will receive blessings such as financial security, but if you choose not to obey other commandments those blessing you would receive from obeying the law of the fast will be of no worth for the rest of your spirit will suffer from your disobedience.

It is then important that in order to receive good health you need to obey the Word of Wisdom and any of the advice of the modern prophets in regards to health. You will not receive these blessings if you disobey the Word of Wisdom which many people do each day and suffer the consequences of poor health.

The Commandments of the Lord

There are many commandments given to us from the Lord, all are important and all are for the benefit of man. It would take volumes of books to examine each and every commandment and the implication on our spiritual health as well as the rest of our health. It is important to note that we must strive to keep and obey all of the commandments of the Lord in order to receive the blessing that come from obedience of those commandments.

There are the commandments in the scriptures that we need to follow, some of them are easy to understand like the ten commandments given to Moses and the children of Israel. There are also the commandments given to the people during the sermon on the Mt. by Jesus. Then there are less known commandments that are extensions of the commandments and things that were written that were changed by modern prophets such as the dietary laws of the Old Testament. It can be very challenging to find all of the commandments in the scriptures and to attempt to interpret and follow each one.

"Jesus said unto him, Thou shalt love the Lord thy God with all they heart, and with all thy soul, and with all thy mind. This is the first and great commandment. And the second is like unto it, Thou shalt love thy neighbor as thyself. On these two commandments hand all the law and the prophets." (Matthew 22:37-40)

To simplify if we will only love God and our neighbor we are obeying all of the commandments. But it is through doing what the Lord says that we show our love for Him, and it is the art of perfecting ourselves and making ourselves better that we are showing our love for God. By loving our neighbor it means that we show compassion, and service for others, and that we do all in our power to the perfecting of the saints. It means that we pray daily to help those in need. It means we do temple work for those who have died. It means that we fulfill our callings in the church to help our neighbors in the church.

We obey the Word of Wisdom because we love our family and want to be around for them and to secure the bond eternal families have. We are breaking the greatest commandments if we choose to harm our bodies, through taking illegal drugs, or we allow ourselves to become lazy and end up relying on the welfare of others.

We must keep in mind the first two great commandments of loving God and loving our neighbor and all other commandments will fall in line and we will be able to receive blessings of health that will help to sustain us in this life to fulfill the mission we were sent here for. In order to fulfill the mission and have blessings of health we need to obey the commandments of God.

The Priesthood of God

"That the rights of the priesthood are inseparably connected with the powers of heaven, and that the powers of heaven cannot be controlled nor handled only upon the principles of righteousness." (D&C 121:36)

The priesthood is the power to act in the name of God, to have the power of heaven given to man to act in Christ's name to fulfill righteous purposes on this earth. In Doctrine and Covenants 121 it goes on to say that a man who has the priesthood will lose it if he has pride and unrighteous dominion. The power of the priesthood is therefore taken away from him if he is unable to obey the commandments of God.

A husband who is abusive to his wife and children will not have the power and blessings of the priesthood in his life. It is only through righteous actions that the priesthood is able to bless the lives of those who are faithful in the gospel. Joseph Smith was able to heal dozens of people who became ill when they first came to Illinois after being driven out of Missouri. Through the priesthood many people were able to become healthy again.

A righteous man who uses his priesthood for righteousness will be strengthened through the priesthood and be able to have good health, yet if he makes the wrong decisions and disobeys the Word of Wisdom or other such commandments then not only will be unhealthy he will lose the spirit and lose the power of the priesthood in his life.

The power of the priesthood can heal people, it can bring people back from the dead, and do amazing things. It can bless people in all aspects of their health including, spiritual, physical, mental, social, and financial. Only both the person giving the priesthood blessing and the one receiving it needs to have faith and be living righteous lives in order for the blessings to come.

Priesthood blessings are intended to be the power of God given to men on earth, and not for the use of men's own desires. This means that even if a righteous man gives a blessing to someone who is also righteous and they both have a lot of faith that the power of the priesthood will heal the person. It might be the will of the Lord that the person does not get better, or that the person and those closest to the person has to go through a challenge or test of faith before the person is healed.

The power of the priesthood also doesn't mean that we can live a life of unhealthy habits and then just get a priesthood blessing to get better. We need to do our part in keeping our bodies and minds healthy, and when we have done all we can do the Lord will then bless us. It could be that a person needs to have a surgery, or take a medicine in order to get better for the time being. If there is a means by a person can get healed through modern medicine, a change in habits, or going to the hospital for medical treatment then the Lord will guide and direct you to do this. Yet if a person is unable to access this the power of the priesthood will be standing by to help assist the recovery of the person.

There are many times when priesthood blessing are necessary and appropriate for a person. Priesthood blessing can be given for a variety of reasons including healing the sick which means physically as well as emotionally sick. A blessing could be given to a child in the form of a father's blessing in order for a child to do better in school, or face a challenge like a mission. Blessings can be given to help a person prepare for things in life like getting a better job, getting an education, and finding someone to get married.

It is always important to know that the priesthood is the power of God to act as if he was here, therefore do not use the priesthood unwisely and hold the blessings of the priesthood as being sacred. The power of the priesthood cannot be used in an unrighteous manner. This is one reason why a person holding the priesthood cannot give himself a blessing.

Provident Living

The church has developed a system of provident living where there are resources for families to start food storage, become financially stable and be able to become self sufficient. It is the goal of the church that all of its members will be able to be self sufficient even in challenging situations like losing employment or a natural disaster.

The welfare of the church is set up so that people will be able to first rely on their own resources, and then their family. If they are unable to do this then they can rely on the church to temporarily help them to get back on their feet. But it is not designed to support someone indefinitely without them working hard to help themselves get out of their need to receive welfare from the church.

Through provident living members of the church learn how to start food storage and to use their food storage, and with food prices these days it would be good to be able to have some food on hand in case food is unavailable at the grocery store or prices are too high. This has happened in several countries causing near panic situations. After the collapse of the Soviet Union, Russia did not have enough food in the grocery stores to feed its people and the prices went through the roof. When McDonalds first opened up in Russia, a meal was worth a week's wages.

Gardening is also encouraged so that members will be able to supplement their food wih food they grow themselves. There are also a lot more benefits to gardening than to eat of the fruit of your labor. There is the exercise and working with nature that helps to invigorate your body and mind.

People in the church are also encouraged to get an education. The Perpetual Education Fund was established for members of the church to be able to get a loan in order to go to college or a technical school. Thousands of members of the church have been able to do this and receive an education thus being able to get out of poverty and help others in their community as well as their families.

The key is to be self sufficient which means to be able to manage your own health and to have healthy habits in your life. It is not the responsibility of the church to do everything for its members. We gain our own salvation through our own actions and not the actions of others. The same goes with our own health. We are in charge of our own health.

Personal Revelation

An important part of our health is through personal revelation. This comes through reading the scriptures, praying, fasting, magnifying our callings, and attending our meetings. I have had a lot of mysteries in my life when it has come to my health. I have gotten sick several times in my life, and one year I was sick twice with about one week apart. I went to the doctor and the doctor said that I had an ulcer and gave me some medicine. This was a temporary fix to something I have been struggling with my entire life.

Every since I was young, I have had stomach pains and nausea, only I was not aware of what it was and thought that it was normal that everyone went through. The only problem was this was not normal and it was a problem that persisted throughout my life, and when I went to the doctor I at least understood what it was that was causing my illness.

But the doctor and the medicine I took did not cure my ulcer, I needed help from the Lord. Through personal revelation and research I was able to find something that help me. I have been able to do several things to control my ulcer and to make my stomach feel a lot better. I have used this same approach on several things in my life relating to my health.

Personal revelation is important for you to be able to figure out many of your health issues. It can help you to be able to develop a plan to lose weight, exercise, or overcome some illness you cannot get rid of. Personal revelation can help you to be able to improve your social health, financial health, and mental health as well.

In order to get personal revelation you need to first have the spirit of the Lord in your life. This often means that you are already living a healthy life and obeying the commandments of the Lord. Then it requires persistence, pondering, fasting, praying, and diligence in seeking the thing you are seeking.

There have been several times when I have been able to get personal revelation through the books that I have read. Often it comes through a thought in my mind or an impression which I search the library for books, and then they books I read give me the answers I need to resolve my issue. I have received revelation through dreams, through word or impressions that come to my mind, and through other people. There have been times when the Lord has given me the answer without me even knowing it, or that I have received an answer to my prayer and only release this much later.

While I was on my mission, I was concerned that I would not be able to exercise enough to maintain my health. At the time I wanted to be a body builder and before my mission I had gained a lot of muscle that I did not want to lose. But I wanted to be a good missionary and to serve the Lord like I should. I prayed for a long time for the answer as I attempted to develop a routine I could follow.

During a Zone conference the general authority who was assigned to the mission was giving a talk when he stopped and paused for a time. He then said, "I am giving this to one of you as an answer to your prayer." He then answered my prayer and comforted me in knowing that the Lord had my back when it came to my health as I served the Lord. I also had lost over fifty pounds the first three months. I got very sick with a bad cold, bloody noses, sore throat, and bad headache. I got a priesthood blessing from some of the missionaries and felt like I would get better and everything would work out. I got better, and wasn't sick the rest of my mission and was able to maintain my health and then when I got back from my mission had a different perspective on my health.

It is only through personal revelation that you will be able to overcome health problems and finds way for you do be healthy. Instead of seeking fad diets and passing exercise routines, seek the advice of the Lord and he will not lead you astray. No one knows you better than your Heavenly Father and with his infinite wisdom will be able to help you have optimum health.

Free Will

"…for behold, ye are free; ye are permitted to act for yourselves…" (Helaman 14:30)

It is this free will also known as free agency that often gets us into trouble. But it also helps us to be able to learn from our mistakes and be able to overcome our weaknesses. It is what makes us stronger and makes us healthier in the long run. But through our free will we can make the wrong decisions in our life that could lead to bad relationships, an unsteady mind, and poor physical and spiritual health. Yet if it wasn't for our agency we would not know what being healthy was like. If we were without getting cold or sick we would not know what it would be like to be happy and healthy.

It is also through the free will of others that we have poor health choices and our environment is polluted. The best thing for each of us is to use our free will to improve our health and the health of others. We are in charge of our own health and our own fate. It is through our own action we are able to exercise, eat right, and work on improving the health of others in our life. If we choose to be smoke, not exercise, or allow our lives to be too stressful we become unhealthy and it is only through our actions that we will be able to stop smoking, start exercising, and reduce the stress in our lives.

We are in charge of our health and even though people and the Lord can help us with our health, in the end it is up to us to be healthy. Health is a matter of choices and actions. It is what we eat, how active we are, and what we think that contributes to our health. There are times when the actions of others may affect our health, but the bulk of our health is the result of what we do in our lives.

Other Religious Ideas

It is important to note some of the other religious ideas here, because some of their ideas in regards to health are important when looking at spiritual health. These ideas are universal truths that have been neglected by western religions, and may even be looked at more or less as philosophy than religion. It is the eastern religious thoughts that are just as important when it comes to spiritual health and bridges the gap between spiritual, physical, and mental health.

When looking at eastern religions we look at the influence first of Hinduism which is one of the oldest traditional religions in the world. It predates the birth of Christ by over a thousand years. Much of its teaching comes from the Vedas which were written in Sanskrit and ancient writing in India.

Hinduism is not what we would think of as an organized religion, because the followers of Hinduism had thousands of different Gods with three or four main Gods. Hindus will pray to their Gods and go to Hindu shrines and temples, but there is no set form of worship or church that they go to. There are certain holy men they may seek advice from and they will make a journey to the River Ganges to bath in its sacred waters, and they will eat a more vegetarian diet.

Much of what Hindus practice such as diet, and daily actions are from Yoga. The way a lot of westerners see Yoga is people sitting in the lotus position meditating. But Yoga is much more than just asanas or poses and meditation. Yoga is a way of life which involves the diet, poses, meditation, and the way you treat others which involves karma and your station in life which is dharma. Yoga means union or harmony, and the practice of Yoga is to bring your life in harmony with everything around you. Through the practice of Yoga you bring your life in balance and in harmony with everything around you. This is done using the spirit to connect everything together.

In Yoga there is the prana which is the breath that brings energy to the body. It is through the breath that energy is brought to the rest of the body. In scientific terms it is the chemical process at which our body converts the oxygen we breathe in to carbon dioxide which makes energy. The greatest amount of energy our body gets is through the air we breathe, not the food we eat. This is why people are able to run marathons, it is also how people can go without food for several days and still be alive.

People who have lung problems and are unable to breathe properly have significantly less energy than those who can breathe normally. It is why athletes who spend their time learning how to breathe efficiently have a lot of energy compared to those who do not exercise. It is the added oxygen we breathe while we exercise that will heat up the body and gives us more energy.

The next time you exercise not the change between your body temperature, and the energy we have. It has to do with the body's movement and the oxygen that is breathed in. Eat a big meal and see how you feel after wards. Chances are you will have less energy after you eat then you did before you ate, because it takes a significant amount of energy to digest the food you ate, and it takes the body a lot of energy to process the food and transport the nutrients around the body. Whereas the conversion process of oxygen is almost spontaneous.

You may even find that by eating less food, and concentrating on breathing better will give you more energy than packing the calories. The key is to be able to breathe properly and allow the energy to flow through your body. This is done through breathing exercises and meditation. The breathing is belly breathing, or allowing the breath to go done below the navel and has the stomach rise and fall with each breath.

The practice of Yoga with breathing, meditation, and correct poses will allow the energy to flow through the body and maintain a balance or harmony in the body. This is why a lot of people are turning to Yoga as a means for achieving ultimate health. There are a lot of benefits for doing Yoga. The great thing about this is that as members of the church we can reap the benefits of Yoga and learn about this ancient form of the balance of the body, spirit, and mind without compromising our faith in the gospel. We do not have to become a Hindu in order to practice Yoga.

When you study Yoga, you will find that even though it has spiritual ties it is not a religion in itself, and you are not worshiping false Gods. You are simply getting in touch with your inner self, your spirit, and connecting it with your mind and body. Just like with anything in the world there are a lot of benefits from Yoga, but if you were to become obsessed with it, and go to more extremes like some people then it could go against the teaching of the church. It is important to be careful when practicing anything that might have contradictory practices to the church.

It is the meditation and the concentration of the breathe and getting in touch with your spirit that is important along with allowing the poses to help with the concentration and to be able to involve the movement of the body. By doing this you will be able to recognize when your body is out of balance and learn how to help bring it back into balance.

The teachings of Hinduism was transformed into Buddhism by Siddhartha Gautahama who was considered the first Buddha or one who is awake. Siddhartha was born in Northern India as a prince. He was privileged and sheltered from the truth of the troubles of life by his father who wanted him to be a great ruler to replace him. Siddhartha was married and being trained to be a ruler when he went among the people and saw a sick person, an old person, and a person who had died. He was so moved by what he saw that he left his family and the palace to find out answers to life.

Siddhartha went out and fasted and meditated on these things when he became awake or enlightened to the truth of life's existence and how suffering is a constant in life and how suffering comes from the desire to posses things, and to overcome desire would end the suffering which would bring about happiness. These are known as the four noble truths. In order to be able to end suffering there are eight things a Buddha must do in order to be able to achieve enlightenment and end suffering. These are known as the eight fold path. In the eight fold path is the way Buddhists achieve nirvana or enlightenment. Part of the eight fold path is meditation which resembles Yoga and what Hindus believe.

The teachings of Buddhism spread throughout Asia and has been transformed into a way of life in China,

Korea, Japan, and Southeast Asia. It is very similar to Hinduism in the fact that it is more of a way of life than a religion. No one worships the Buddha or any God in Buddhism. Siddhartha was asked if he was a God, prophet, or messenger of God, and he replied that he was just a man who was awake. According to Buddhism anyone who is awake to the truths of life is a Buddha.

Presently the Dali Lama is considered a Buddha and spends his time teaching people about the four noble truths, the eight fold path, and living a peaceful life. His people do not worship him, but see him as a reincarnation of a Buddhist monk or Dali Lama in Tibet. There are several different points of practice in which as LDS would not fall in line with the gospel like reincarnation and it is important to look at Buddhism in a proper perspective and to again look at the art of meditation and coming to a balance of the mind, spirit, and body.

In China the idea of the body's energy has come to be known as chi, has been a standard for Chinese medicine for centuries. It involved the movement of chi through slow movements known as tai chi, the meditation and breathing known as chi kong, and also includes herbal medicine and acupuncture or acupressure. The basic concept came from Buddhism which came from Yoga. It is also part of Confucianism, and Taoism. Many of the same principals connect with many of the eastern religions. Just like how Abraham is the main connection among all of the western religions.

Studying eastern medicine, thought, and practice the common theme or principle is the idea of an inner source of power or energy in which we can control. It is important to keep this energy in balance with our lives or we have poor health. There are a lot of practices to keep this energy or spirit in balance with our bodies and minds and to connect all aspects of our health together. These practices involve Yoga, tai chi, chi chong, and meditation. By doing these things we can achieve this balance which is represented with the Ying Yang symbol.

The Ying Yang symbol represents balance or harmony and teaching another important principle of the idea that everything has its opposite, and that there is opposition in all things. This is an important truth and aspect of our lives that will help us understand health a little better and how we need to balance our lives. If health was just a matter of exercise then we would just exercise, and if exercise brought about good health, then the more exercise we did the healthier we become, but this is not the case there must be a balance in all the things we do.

"For it must needs be, that there is an opposition in all things. If not so, my first-born in the wilderness, righteousness could not be brought to pass, neither wickedness, neither holiness nor misery, neither good nor bad. Wherefore, all things must needs be a compound in one; where-fore, if it should be one body it must needs remain as dead, having no life neither death, nor corruption nor incorruption, happiness nor misery, neither sense nor insensibility." (2 Nephi 2:11)

The ancient wisdom of the gospel can be found in fragments in other eastern religions. With the light of Christ many good people through history have come up with sound ideas that work in obtaining overall health. Following the gospel and the teaching of modern day prophets is the most important part of spiritual health, and there is also wisdom in Eastern thought that will help aid spiritual health and help to connect to the other forms of health.

Armor of God

"Put on the whole armor of God, that ye may be able to stand against the wiles of the devil." (Ephesians 6:11)

Satan would have all of us fall into temptation and to destroy our spiritual health and thus destroying the rest of our health. It is important to take on the armor of God to be able to withstand the evils around us. Society may be conscious of being healthy through diet, exercise, and living healthier including doing things for the environment. But when it comes to spiritual health society does not promote living a more Christ like life.

Church is something that is separated from the rest of our lives instead of being part of it. Many people believe in some form or morality, but this too can be distorted in how many people believe that it is okay to do what you want just as long as you are not directly hurting other people. The sanctity of marriage and the family have gone under attack and more families are destroyed and children are living in single parent situation with their parents living with a partner without the trust and commitment of marriage.

The entire concept of living spiritually has been lost among the masses. There are some glimmers of hope especially among the members of the church who promote a spiritual lifestyle that is recognized by others. But there is Satan and his followers who would have people believe that they do not have to be spiritual to be healthy, and if you want to be spiritual you can just live how you want just as long as you promote peace and tolerance of others.

It talks in Ephesians about having loins girt about with truth and a breastplate of righteousness. We need to have truth in our lives and watch out for false things like the idea that you can live a spiritual life without having to go to church. In order to fill our lives with truth and righteousness we need to keep the gospel in our lives and participate fully in the church. In Ephesians it also talks about the shield of faith and the sword of the Spirit. In order to withstand the temptation of Satan and to be able to have good spiritual health we need to have faith, and practice those things we have been taught to do in the gospel.

It is through being spiritually healthy that we are able to be able to withstand the temptations of Satan and be able to live a healthy happy life. The foundation starts with spirituality and it connects to all other aspects of health.

King Benjamin who was a righteous king in the Americas said to his people, "…I am like as yourselves, subject to all manner of infirmities in body and mind; yet I have been chosen by this people, and consecrated by my father, and was suffered by the hand of the Lord that I should be a ruler and a king over this people; and have been kept and preserved by his matchless power, to serve you with all the might, mind and strength which the Lord hath granted unto me." (Mosiah 2:11)

He mentioned that he was just like the people of his kingdom and was afflicted both in his body and mind, meaning that he struggled with health issues just like those he ruled over. But that it was because of the Lord and his spiritual health that sustained him so that he could serve his people and help them. It is through spiritual health that we can gain the strength to overcome physical and mental challenges in our lives.

"And the Spirit giveth light to every man that cometh into the world; and the Spirit enlighteneth every man through the world, that hearkeneth to the voice of the Spirit." (D&C 84:46)

We all have spirits, and are given the light of Christ in our lives, and those of us who are baptized in the church also receive the Holy Ghost. All of this means that we are spiritual being surrounded by the help of the heavens and are given these blessings of the Spirit if we only listen to the Spirit and keep the Spirit in our lives it will guide us in the way we should go which is to having a balance in our lives bringing about overall health.

To Do List

1. Keep prayer part of your daily routine. You should include gratitude, repentance, and humility with each prayer.
2. Keep the commandments of the Lord including the Word of Wisdom, and being happy.
3. Be worthy to attend the temple, and attend the temple when you are able.
4. Attend all your church meetings and make the effort to listen to the Holy Ghost and learn from every lesson and talk given.
5. Read and study the scriptures daily making it part of your daily routine and take the time to ponder and pray about what you read.
6. Fulfill your church callings and magnify them in the sense that you put forth the effort to do your best in the calling you have accepted.
7. Pay a full tithe and fast offerings each month.
8. Fast once a month making sure to pray and study the scriptures as you fast.
9. Keep a journal at least once a week and record the things you did that week and bear your testimony in it.
10. Make sure to fulfill your responsibilities in your family by having prayers, reading the scriptures, having family home evening, family council, eating together, and doing family activities together on a weekly basis.

Chapter Four: Mental Health

"For as he thinketh in his heart, so is he..."
(Proverbs 23:7)

The next part of health is the mind. If a person doesn't have a healthy mind he will not have a healthy body. The mind is the command center to the body. If the brain is damaged it will affect the body. It sends messages to the body to be able to breathe, have the heart beat, and the muscles contract. When the nerves that are message relays to the body are injured it breaks the communication between the brain and those parts of the body that can no longer receive messages from the brain.

The brain is a complex organ of the body that is not fully understood by the medical community. It is said that we only use about ten percent of our brains which leaves a lot of room for speculation as to the functions of the brain. What we do know is that the brain serves as the control center of the entire body and its functions. It is also affected by environmental stimulus sent to the brain from the sense of touch, sight, smell, taste, and hearing. These senses send stimulus such as a hot stove from the touch of a finger to the brain in the response as pain and the reaction of removal of the finger of the stove.

The stimulus we receive from our senses causes chemical reactions to occur in the brain in turn creates an emotion, the emotion then create thoughts, which brings about an action. All of this is done faster than the speed of light, but can be altered by a number of things like how the thoughts might be formulated or other stimulus affecting the emotions. In any given moment we might have dozens of different stimulus going to the brain. Then there is the sixth sense or intuition which we can refer to our spiritual side that will also influence our emotions and thoughts.

It is like the captain of the Starship Enterprise receiving all of the stimulus of what is happening around him. He is the brain of the ship, and the crew are the emotions that the stimulus creates as well as the thoughts. Once he gets advice from his thoughts he makes an informed decision. This can further be illustrated by the personality of the different members of the crew with Ricker being impulsive, Counselor Troy being compassionate and being able to sense the emotions of others, Data with his analytical advice to the captain, and Worf with his courage to face fears.

In all of us we have the same crew of emotions to help us to navigate the stars and vanquish our enemies. It just takes a lifetime of experience and learning to be able to develop a good process of thinking that leads to the right decisions in our lives and making doing the right actions.

In essence our brains gather information through our senses including our spiritual sense. We have emotions that help us to formulate thoughts, and then we make a decision based on our thoughts and then take action. This can be very fast, or it may be very slow depending on our experiences in our lives and what we are presented with. Then there is also the temptations that flood our minds on a moment by moment basis. These temptations are intended to confuse us and to have us make the wrong decision. Satan will use false emotions to influence our thoughts and actions.

With all of these things come at our brains at a time it isn't any wonder we have a difficult time making decisions in our lives and be able to take the appropriate action. But in order to be healthy we need to have a healthy mind which means that we need to recognize those emotions and thoughts that are beneficial to our lives as well as others in our life. The mind can be susceptible to addictions and habits that can be harmful, some can also be helpful. As an example we might grow accustomed to brushing our teeth as a habit and if we do not brush our teeth we become agitated and disturbed until we brush our teeth. We might also become addicted to a drug or bad habit and it thus becomes hard to stop the habit which causes a lot of pain and suffering in our lives.

Emotions

Emotions can be seen as being positive and negative such as love, and hate. If we look at our emotions in this way we tend to seek the positive emotions and avoid or get rid of the negative ones. Only this causes us a lot of problems, because if we ignore or avoid certain emotions over other emotions we will not be able to fully understand them and their source.

Fear may be seen as a negative emotion, yet without fear we would do things that would cause us great harm and may cause others to be harmed as well. There is a place for fear in our lives. It is a natural emotion that will illicit a fight or flight response where our body will release adrenaline to prepare us to fight or run away from the potential danger. Only not all fear comes from physical danger. You might experience fear when you have to give a talk in church, or you might be afraid to talk to your parents or someone else in your life. It can be real like a bear coming after you, or it might be perceived that people may make fun of you when you give your talk in church. In one case fear is warning you that a bear is going to hurt you and you need to do something fast, in the other case it is a false fear that is placed in your mind by Satan to prevent you from giving your talk in church.

There have been times in my life when fear has helped guide me into doing the right thing like being careful around a cliff and avoiding a group of people who are about to get into a fight. It has also prevented me from accomplishing a lot of things in my life, like being able to talk to people and tell them how I feel or some of the desires of my heart. Satan has placed fear as an obstacle in my life that has caused me to not do something that I needed to do. If I would have given in to my fears, I would have never been able to have graduated from college, went on a mission, or gotten married. It was only through faith that I was able to overcome my fears and do the things I needed to do in life.

So when looking at fear, you have to understand that it is both a positive and negative emotion. It is a powerful emotion and this is something Satan uses to force us to not do things we need to do and avoid things that are helpful to others. Many people avoid serving people because they are afraid that the people they serve will not want them to. So it is important to exam fear you have in your life, and make a decision if it is positive and is a warning that something is wrong like you are being abused by a friend, or negative that you are afraid to do something that would help you and others around you.

If you are experiencing emotions like fear that are preventing you from attending college, asking someone on a date, or applying for a job. It is important to recognize this and have faith in the Lord to give you the courage to overcome those fears and do what you need to do in life to improve it. This is a big part of the learning process in life to overcome your fears.

Emotions that are thought of as being positive can also be turned into something that is negative. There are a lot of bad things done in the name of love. A person might become obsessed with another person because they love them, and cannot live without them. Initial love is a response to a lot of different stimulus and chemical reactions in the brain which make us feel good, only these things are temporary. It is important to understand that if you are attracted to a person it is not true love, but your hormones are making you feel good being around the person, which you might be thinking this is love.

Satan is a master at making people believe they are in love with a person, or that the spirit is telling them that the person they are seeing is the one and only, the love at first sight thing that is part of our fairytales. The reality is that this feeling of love is only temporary, and then once we get to know the person and our pleasure chemicals calm down we are then able to see the true person we thought we loved. This is why it is important not to rush into relationships. Yet Satan can use this as an opportunity to persuade people not to get into relationships and to wait too long to get married or have children. It is important to pray and seek out the spirit to give you personal revelation on the matter.

Love, happiness, and many of the other so called good emotions can be great motivators to do good. They can help us to come up with thoughts that we can use to make informed decisions. Emotions can be great guides to our life in how we should live, only we have to understand them and understand the meaning behind them.

If you are experiencing hate towards someone it would not do you any good to try and avoid the feelings you are experiencing without first understanding them. You need to ask yourself why you are made at the person and hate them. Then you can start thinking about how you can get rid of the hate you have for the person. Often emotions are combinations of other emotions you have. You might hate someone because you are afraid that the person will get promoted over you at work, or the person might steal away someone you care for, or the person has something you really want which brings in envy.

Once you have examined your emotions and understand them you can dismiss them easier, and work toward overcoming them and replace them with other more positive emotions. Then once an emotion crosses the stage in your mind you can step back from it and examine it then replace it with another emotion or come up with thoughts that are productive.

Thoughts

Emotions bring thoughts in our minds. Some of those thoughts are temptations form Satan and his followers tempting you to do something you will regret later. We are what we think. Many of our actions are the direct result of our thoughts. If we think it we will do it. This is why it is important to fill you mind with wholesome righteous thoughts.

My daughter told me I was stupid on day while we were on vacation. I got upset with her and later when I was talking to her. I asked her, "Why did you say that to me?"

She said, "I don't know, I just thought about it and then did it."

This is often the case, we think about something and then we do it. It might be a word, or an action, but if the word or action is from Satan then there are negative consequences. If it is a positive thought then the outcome is often positive. But before we do or say anything we first think about it. If we do not step back and examine those thoughts then they may cause us harm. This is a great teaching experience to have thoughts and to take a step back and examine those thoughts to determine what the consequence will be if we take action on those thoughts.

Just like with emotions we can see the thoughts come across the stage of our mind and be able to replace them at will. It is important not to let negative thoughts and emotions to take root, because then they will dominate the stage of our mind and become overgrown pushing out all of the positive emotions and thoughts in our minds. This is why people who become depressed are often not very rational and believe in false notions like no one likes them and they are no good. If a thought is nourished with time and allowing it to grow it will dominate our minds. Just like an addictive substance a thought or emotion can be just as addictive and damaging as an illegal drug.

People who are depression may find it comforting to be depressed and will resist the attempt by others to get out of depression. They may believe that there is no such thing as happiness, and they find safety in feeling sorry for themselves. I experienced this in my life, and it is not a good place to be. It is okay to have thoughts of helping others, saying the right words, and standing up to bullies, but even these should have a limit on the stage of our mind so that we can be receptive to the promptings of the Holy Ghost when there is a dangerous situation in our life, or that we are suppose to be serious about our work, or schooling.

Like what was spoken of in the previous chapter it is important to have a balance in your mind and to recognize those thoughts and emotions that you should not dwell on and allow them to grow. There are obvious thoughts that we should not allow to grow in our minds like anything that is harmful to ourselves or others, things that will be against the will of the Lord. It is important to know the difference between those thoughts and emotions that are form Satan and those that are from the Lord. One simple tool to use is that all good things come from God and all bad things come from Satan. It is your job to distinguish between those things that are good and those things that are bad.

Desire

"I know that he granteth unto men according to their desire…" (Alma 29:4)

Desire is the most powerful motivator to get things done. It is what compels people to do the things they do for both evil and good. A criminal who commits a crime first had a thought or temptation and then developed a desire to do the crime. Desire is also what causes people a lot of pain and sorrow.

If you desire to be with someone, but that person doesn't desire to be with you it causes a lot of pain. This is why most of the violence in the United States is around domestic violence that involved desire to posses someone who does not want to be possessed. You might even have a desire to get a job, and when you do not get it there is sorrow, or it might be that your desire is to have a big house or a nice car, but you are unable to obtain these things because of your financial situation and therefore you become depressed and envious to those who have those things.

Desire can be used for bad or good depending on our intent. Satan can have us desire many things that do harm to others, or that is impossible for us to have thus causing a lot of sorrow. It is the attachment to the things we desire and the obsession that can cause a lot of harm. We need to focus our desires on righteous purposes and understand that life is filled with unfulfilled desires and that if we do not reach our goals we move on and if those goals are worthy enough we find another way to achieve them.

It is through desire we can be motivated and persisted with achieving something of great worth. If we did not have desire in our lives it would be hard to do anything, we would become depressed and bored with life unwilling to do anything because of the lack of desire to get out of bed and take the first step for the day.

In Buddhism and Eastern thought they believe in eliminating desire from our lives. To some extent this is correct in the fact that we need to have the proper intent and the right perspective on our desire. There is nothing wrong to have an underlining desire to help people and to preach the gospel. But if we allow our desire to become distorted to the fact that we destroy our lives attempting to help others and neglect our family because we have a desire to be with those who are less fortunate more than with our family, also it could be that we may not have an opportunity to directly help other people for a while and if we are attached to this desire we may become distraught with the lack of opportunities.

It might be that you are unable to go on a mission, or that when you retire you want to go on a mission with your wife, only she is unable to go on a mission for medical concerns and you start resenting your wife because you are unable to go on a couple mission. All of these desires can be distorted to the point that they are causing more bad than good.

But if you have a desire to help others and find several small ways to help people and focus on those you are most involved with such as your family, friends, home teaching families, you will be able to do a lot of good with this intent or desire. The same would go with preaching the gospel. You do not have to go on a mission to preach the gospel and it is better to start with those you know are not members of the church first and this will give you the greatest joy.

Desire can be a great motivator and it is important to take a step back now and then and look at our desires to see if they are in line with God's will and are of benefit to yourself and others around you. It is the desires of our hearts that we are judged on, and it is our desires that will lead us to do things as well. The wicked among us have evil intentions and desires, and the righteous have good intentions and desires.

It is through our intentions and desires we are able to accomplish a lot of our goals and define who we are. If we intend or desire to do good, good will come our way. This is also known in Eastern thought as Karma. What we do will come back to us, starting with our desires.

Knowledge and Wisdom

When we think about mental health knowledge and wisdom is one of the first things we think about. Some people would say that geniuses have healthy minds, and those who do not have much intelligence has a weaker or unhealthy mind. It is important to be able to seek knowledge and wisdom and it does help to improve the mental function of the brain. Those who have kept their brains more active in life are less likely to get Alzheimer's disease.

Alzheimer's disease is the ultimate brain killer. It slowly destroys all functions of the brain to the point the person doesn't know who they are and cannot recognize anyone else. It is a terrible disease that has a huge impact on the family. It is hard to watch as your father or mother forgets who you are and their grandchildren. Alzheimer's disease is in the top ten killers in America and is rising each year.

The question is how do we obtain knowledge and wisdom? How much do we need? Are there people who are limited in the knowledge they can have? We are all different when it comes to knowledge and wisdom and learning. Not is our capacity and speed at which we learn is different, our own free will comes into play with this as well. We are able to choose what and when we learn things. This is why so many children struggle each year in school, because some are ready and willing to learn, while there are many who are not ready and not willing to learn.

It is said that when a student is ready there will be a teacher. Unfortunately we have things reversed and attempt to force children to learn on a structured schedule and curriculum. This is great for about 20 percent of the population, but for the remaining 80 percent they struggle and many of them drop out of school.

Obtaining knowledge is a lifelong mission for all of us. Even till the day we die we are learning and growing, and it is our responsibility to look for learning opportunities. It doesn't meant that we have to go to school for the rest of our life. Some people find that they like going to school to learn things, but a lot of learning can take place in our homes and at church. This is why members of the church start giving talks in primary and continue to give talks throughout their lives, and it is why all members of the church have callings. It is through our experiences in the church and fulfilling our callings that we do a great deal of learning and growing. Most members of the church are called to a calling that they have never had before and learn a great deal by fulfilling the calling.

In the family there are a lot of learning experiences taking place from childhood through to parenthood. This is why it is important that parents are able to spend a lot of quality teaching time with their children. This means that parents are reading scriptures with their children, saying prayers, having family home evening, gardening with their children, teaching children to be responsible through chores and giving them an allowance so that they can learn to pay their tithing.

Often learning takes place by example. Children love to do what adults do, because they want to be like them. They will observe the adults and older children in their lives and mimic their behavior thus learning what others do around them. This is important that children have good role models of both adults and older children in their lives.

Learning is a self guided journey through life. My mother tried to force me to read every night to her in elementary school and so I had hated to read books. Until I started to read books I liked, and heard about how popular writers read over a hundred books a year, so then I got started on reading a lot of books, and now read over a hundred books a year. Many of them are audio books I listen to, and some of them are children's books, but I have learned a great deal from the different books I have read. In fact I believe I have learned a great deal from the books I have read then all of the classes in school that I have taken.

I have also learned that I am able to learn a great deal more according to my desire to learn something and the challenge that is involved in the learning experience. When I went through getting my black belt in taekwondo, I learn so much more than I did getting my master's degree. I also learned a lot while I was backpacking in the Absorka Mountains in Wyoming more than I learned while attending an entire semester at college.

It is important to learn a variety of things in your life, and to have a desire and compassion to learn certain things in your life and become a specialist in these areas. You can learn a great deal going through different experiences as well. This is why a lot of people are able to learn a great deal from learning something different such as another language, a musical instrument, learning to rock climb, scuba dive, or fly a plan. Everything in life that has a little risk to it is worthwhile to learn.

It is important to be careful and not jump into something that is over your head and find yourself in trouble. When I went sky diving, I went to a mini class at first and from qualified instructors learned what I needed to do and went with an instructor and jumped out of a perfectly good airplane with the instructor tandem meaning that I was attached to the instructor and he was there to help if I needed help.

Seek out knowledge through books, classes, internet, and your experiences. Make life fun and exciting through learning new things. Let the adventure begin. The knowledge and wisdom you can have is endless and there is no limit to the brains capacity to knowledge. Become eager to learn new things and humble enough to know that you need to continue to learn things throughout the rest of your life.

When I was in elementary school, I couldn't wait to get into junior high and high school. I thought that once I graduated from high school, I would not have to learn another thing. Then when I was attending college, I thought that when I graduated I would not have to learn anything else. I also thought that after my mission and after I went through the temple that my spiritual learning would be complete, then I got married and had to raise children.

One thing I have learned is that there is no end to learning and growth it is one constant in life and through eternity that we can look forward to. It is those who do not know this or refuse to understand this who are stopped in their progression. You look at people who have an attitude that they do not want to learn new things and are unwilling to attempt to learn things who suffer the consequences of poverty, depression, and mental illness. Often times it is not the mental illness that is preventing the ability to learn. It is the lack of wanting to learn that leads to mental illness. People in this state of being lack the proper motivation in life to want to learn.

The first week of my classes I know which students will fail the class and which ones will get a good grade. It has to the positive attitude and the willingness to learn. Teachers cannot force their students to learn. Students need to want to learn first. When the student is willing to learn there will always be a teacher. The teacher might be from school, a parent, a friend, a primary teacher, or even a stranger.

Meditation and Memorization

Mental health is all about keeping the mind active, this can be done through learning things as well as through mental exercises like solving problems, memorization, and meditation. These three things will keep your mind active and clear. Things like video games, television, and idle thoughts can lead to an unclear mind full of confusing thoughts and images. I know from personal experience that having idle thoughts that do not have any meaning or negative thoughts can lead down a path you do not want your mind to go.

You can memorize just about anything and keep that in your mind repeating it daily or weekly to keep it in your mind. I have been involved in both primary and scouts for several years and it is necessary in primary to have memorized the 13 Articles of Faith. In Scouts it is the oath, law, slogan, motto, and outdoor code along with Leave No Trace and a number of knots. The knots are important because not only do scouts have to memorize how to do a knot it is tactile which gives more connections in the brain. Those who practice basketball or other sports doing drills over and over again are memorizing how to do something perfect. It is a lot like juggling where you need to learn how to throw the balls in the air in the right way in order to catch them.

There are a lot of things you can memorize some out of necessity like all of your phone numbers, addresses, and passwords. Then there are things that can be useful and good for the mind such as scriptures or hymns that can help to replace unwholesome thoughts in your mind when the time comes and you are tempted with those thoughts. There are a lot of great quotes out there you can memorize as well that can keep your mind on the straight and narrow.

In taekwondo, I memorized other phrases that talked about the proper actions and thoughts that a true warrior should have like, "having might for right, and only using martial art skills to protect the weak and innocent, and never to harm others." The martial arts training I have had, taught me how to meditate which is great to be able to think properly.

Meditation is simply concentrating on something. You are meditating when you watch a movie, listen to music, read a book, or text a friend. This does not mean that all meditation is good for you, in fact Satan has used meditation as a way to distract us from doing things we should be doing. As an example, I have heard of teenagers texting friends until two o'clock in the morning. This is unhealthy, and texting too much is unhealthy it prevents a person from enjoying life and doing other things in their life, like doing homework, reading a book, doing fun activities like rock climbing, dancing, or having family home evening.

The reason why it is important to meditate is to be able to recharge the mind and reset it on the right path. If someone is spending a lot of time texting, playing video games, or listening to music, then his mind will be focused on those things and it will be difficult for him to be able to concentrate on other more important things. Through proper meditation the mind will be more focused and clear. Solving problems with become easier, and listening to the Holy Ghost will be so much easier as well. The Holy Ghost will not be with you when you are watching a movie unless it is an inspirational movie.

The first thing to do when meditating is to find a place and time when you can meditation without interruptions or distractions. If you cannot set aside five minutes or find a place without interruptions or distractions then you have a problem and you need to resolve it before you attempt to meditate. Then you need to start out with the most basic form of mediation where you concentrate on your breathing through your nose called belly breathing because your stomach rises and falls with each breathe.

You are breathing slowly and deeply with each breath allowing it to fill your lungs and concentrating on feeling the breathe enter and exit the body. You will want to do this several times before you attempt any other form of meditation. Breathing meditation is something you can always come back to when you want to and you can do it just about any time you feel the need to meditate. You could do it when you are in a traffic jam, at school during a test to get more focused on the test questions. This form of meditation is also critical in helping you breathe better which has several other benefits such as more energy, and increased overall health.

Other forms of meditation you can try can be just starting out with breathing meditation and then moving your chi or energy around your body. You can even concentrate on lowering your heart rate, and focusing on different parts of your body such as those areas you might be sore or feel pain in. You can practice clearing the stage of your mind so that you have no thoughts going across the stage and that you mind is completely clear without any thoughts.

Sensory meditation is also very powerful. This is where you use your senses for meditation. You can listen to a noise like a bell, music, or a chant to meditate. You could look at the flickering light of a candle, or an object to focus on to clear your mind. There is also smell, and touch in the form of acupressure or massage that can be part of meditation. Then there is taste. You might ask yourself when was the last time you actually tasted your food? In America we tend to eat to quickly and do not savor the food we eat.

Food meditation alone will help you control your diet, lose weight, and digest your food better. It is simply slowing down when you eat and really tasting what you put in your mind. When you do this it is important not to eat too many sweets, or foods that are too spicy, because then it is hard to be able to pick out the small hints of taste in the food you eat.

You can practice mediation in almost everything you do, it simply requires slowing down and focusing more on what you are doing. So when you take a walk you are feeling the breeze in your face, smelling the flowers you pass by, feeling the ground you are walking on, listening to the sounds of the birds and people around you. You can even taste the air around you and know when rain is coming or if you are near salty water like in the ocean. Things will start to come alive for you and you will be amazed at what you will experience. It will be like waking up from a dream.

Through meditation you will be able to think more clearly, perform your tasks better, be able to listen to the Holy Ghost and those around you better, and be able to have better mental health. Meditation has been used by Satan ever since the beginning of time to distract people and lead them down the wrong path in life. It is important that you do not allow this to happen and use meditation to be able to focus on what is the most important things in life.

"For it came to pass after I had desired to know the things that my father had seen, and believing that the Lord was able to make them known unto me, as I sat pondering in mine heart I was caught away in the Spirit of the Lord, yea, into an exceedingly high mountain, which I never had before seen, and upon which I never had before set my foot." (1 Nephi 11:1)

Nephi pondered the things his father had told him, or in other words he meditated on the words his father had said to him and desired to know more about those things. Because of this Nephi was able to have the desire of his heart and learn of what his father had said to him. Prayer and meditation is often what it takes to receive answers to prayers and get personal revelation. Prayer is also a form of meditation where we are concentrating on communication to the Lord.

Reflection and Mindfulness

"But, behold, I say unto you, that you must study it out in your mind; then you must ask me if it be right, and if it is right, I will cause that your bosom shall burn within you; therefore, you shall feel that it is right." (D&C 9:8)

You should reflect upon everything you do in life in order to be able to be guided by the Holy Ghost in doing the right things. The more you reflect on things and study them out in your mind the more you will be able to make informed decisions and be guided by the Holy Ghost in what you do. This can be done in the form of writing a journal and reflecting on the things you have done every week, and taking the time to reflect on the things you have done each day. I have used the time before I go to bed to reflect on the day and to use that reflection in my prayer before I end the day and go to bed.

Mindfulness is the simple art of being mindful or aware of what is happening around you. It is the ability to exam what is happening at the present moment. Being mindful is simply living in the present. We often get caught up in day dreaming about the future or thinking about how it would be wonderful to get a wonderful job, house, and car. But dwelling upon the future can become a huge distraction just like watching too much television can do. We also may dwell on the past and become depressed thinking about all of our failures or mistakes we have made, or thinking about a time when we were doing better. It is okay to remember the past and even learn from it, but it can be damaging to focus on the past.

You need to live in the present and be aware of what is happening right now. Just like I am concentrating on my writing this book, I am aware of what my thoughts are as I write the book. If I were to think of the future or the past then my thoughts would wonder and it would be hard to be able to write this book. It is called writers block, because the writer is thinking too much about the future or the past and is not in the present to come up with the right words to put on the paper. By living in the present you can secure positive outcomes for the future, and you cannot do anything about the past, because it has already happened and you cannot change it.

Mental Illness

Mental illnesses can be caused by a variety of things like heredity where someone is born with it, it could be caused by exposure to some environmental factor such as abusive parents, or a dramatic event like fighting in a war. It can also be caused by a toxic chemical introduced to the brain, or a dramatic head injury. The lack of oxygen to the brain can cause brain damage as well as a child being shaken hard. The key to all of these illnesses is prevention, taking the precaution to wear a helmet when you ride a bike, avoiding using drugs, being careful with children, and preparing for a personal crisis you know is going to happen.

There are mental illnesses that are irreversible and there is nothing that can be done about them, and then there are others that are treated through medication. Then there are mental illnesses that are treated through therapy. Psychology is a relatively young science and many of the practices are argued over. Even insurance companies often do not recognize therapy as medical treatment.

Through the years mental illness has been treated as something other than part of health. I remember a woman saying that her brother who was mentally challenged was possessed with the devil. Mental illness has often been misunderstood and often mistreated with people being shut away in an asylum and treated like outcastes being doped up and even used as human test subjects.

The human brain is a complex organ that can do amazing things, but can also break down without warning. Some people can go through horrifying experiences and be able to rise above them and function normally, whereas some people might be exposed to minor stressful situations and end up cracking. There is some evidence that mental health is hereditary with some illnesses, and only slightly in others.

The best way to treat a mental illness would be just like any other illness, do some research on it and then come up with a plan. You might have to see a doctor, and come up with a treatment, or you might be able to just work it out through some basic methods of mental health that has partly been discussed.

The best way to treat minor depression would be to reduce stress in your life, understand that it can be temporary, everyone goes through depression at one point in their life. You can get help from family, friends, and the Lord through prayer. By living healthily spiritually and physically it will help you feel better. It is important to get up every morning and start of the day working hard and continue throughout the day. A big part of depression is not wanting to do anything and not caring about anything. It is important to be active in working hard doing things at home, work, and school, then to work hard at helping and serving others. The best way to overcome feeling sorry for your self is to help others.

The best way to overcome ADD or ADHD would be to eat a healthy diet, be actively involved in several different hobbies and practice meditation techniques. I have ADD and the best way for me to be able to concentrate on things is to channel my energy into things I like and to exercise a lot, being physically active helps to calm the activity in my mind. There are many people especially children are being treated with medication to help this, which could be a blessing for some, but with any medication it is important to monitor it and do not have them use the medication all of the time. ADD and ADHD can be misdiagnosed for those who have it and those who do not, especially with children whose normal hyper activity for their age level could be taken as them having ADHD, or a child who is timid as having ADD.

Doctors are in the business to prescribe drugs, and there are times when a doctor will prescribe a drug that is not necessary. This could result in severe side effects. It is important to always look at several different treatments for an illness and to make an informed decision as to which one is the best for you and your children. It doesn't make sense to spend a lot of money on medications that may have side effects when you can control it through exercise and eating right.

Gratitude

An important part of mental health is gratitude. You cannot be happy without having gratitude. You need to give a prayer of thanks each day, and to thank the Lord for your home, family friends, the clothes you have, the job you have, the experiences you are able to have, and for your health.

It should be a constant in your life, and it will help you to be positive and be able to handle the most difficult situations in your life. With gratitude you will be able to have the proper perspective in live and be able to help others through your gratitude. Those who are not grateful for all that life has to offer them, are often miserable and depressed. They lack the proper perspective and understand about life, and are unable to make things happen in their life. They then start to blame others for their misfortunes when they are often doing it to themselves because it is what they are thinking and their actions are the result of their negative thoughts.

Be grateful and you will receive more blessings that you will have room for, and the gratitude in your life will help to secure a more healthy life one in which you will be even more grateful for. Your gratitude to others will also help your social health as well as the other aspects of your health.

To Do List

1. Do research on mental health
2. Memorize scriptures, poems, hymns, and famous quotes
3. Meditation on a daily basis starting with breathing meditation
4. Pray daily with prayers of thanks, refection on things you have done asking for repentance of the mistakes you have made, and to pray for others.
5. Read my goal each year is to read more than a 100 books
6. Keep things in the proper perspective and do not allow your emotions to control you. Remember to take a step back before you react to a situation.
7. Always be positive and grateful for the things you have. Look for the bright things in life and not the ugly things.
8. Keep a journal and write in it at least once a week about the things that happened during the week. Include spiritual experiences, as well as the good and bad things that happened during the week. Let it help you to reflect on your life and the things that happens to you.
9. Keep physically and spiritually healthy
10. Reduce the stress in your life by eliminating some things, and come up with an effective stress reducing plan such as practicing yoga and exercise.

Chapter Five: Physical Health

"If any man defile the temple of God, him shall God
destroy; for the temple of God is holy, which temple
ye are." (1 Corinthians 3:17)

Our bodies have been given to us as a gift from our
Father in Heaven and are considered temples of God. When
it comes to physical health there are a lot of things to
consider such as; diet, exercise, sleep, and hygiene. There
is also chastity and treating the body as a temple meaning
not doing excessive piercings, getting tattoos, and defacing
the body. Like the passage of scripture above, the Lord will
hold accountable those who defile their bodies which are
holy.

We are in a constant struggle with physical ailments
and challenges in our lives. As pioneers they were in
constant physical danger with disease, struggle with the
environment, and common accidents which today would be
easily treated, but back then where life threatening. Despite
their physical challenges, the pioneers did amazing physical
accomplishments working from sun up to sun down all
week most of their life with the children even working
alongside their parents to farm, ranch, and survive the
environment.

Today we have equally daunting physical
challenges only ours is almost the reverse. We have too
little physical activity and too much food instead of too
little. This has caused an increase in heart disease, cancer,
and diabetes. We are still faced with disease, accidents, and
many other ailments as did our ancestors only we have
better medical care than they did, but we must still face the
challenges of dealing with our bodies and all of the things
that go with them.

Satan has used the temptations of the flesh to his
advantage over us. There are many temptations of the flesh

which can almost be irresistible for many. It is these appetites that compel us to do things we would not normally do. The desires for physical pleasures cause our mind to not think to clearly and may result in doing something we regret later.

The things we do to the body will affect our spiritual and mental health as well. If we allow our physical bodies to be unhealthy then it will be hard for us to perform our church duties and we become depressed, and depression will lead to inactivity in the church and could eventually lead to falling away from the gospel. Many of the people who are mentally and spiritually ill are those who have physical problems as well. They are all connected and just one physical illness or set back in your physical health could bring you down both spiritually and mentally in a heartbeat.

Sleep

"...cease to sleep longer than is needful; retire to thy bed early, that ye may not be weary; arise early, that your bodies and your minds may be invigorated."
(D&C 88:124)

Sleep is essential for health, because it allows the body to recover and rest from working, and it also helps to reduce stress and help to process all of the thoughts and emotions that are flowing through the mind, many of them are unconscious thoughts and emotions that are in our minds. We can feel it when we do not have enough sleep. This is often accompanied by headaches, dizziness, nausea, exhaustion, and inability to think clearly. It could also be accompanied by irritability, combativeness, and hallucinations, this is why when people talk about seeing ghosts, being abducted by aliens, or have psychotic episodes they are just sleep deprived. We need our sleep in order to be healthy.

In America we have poor sleep habits which contributes to insomnia, and in which causes health problems. The first thing would be relate to time. The amount of time one sleeps, and the time a person goes to bed and gets up in the morning. The amount of time a person sleeps depends of the person. On general people need at least 8 hours of uninterrupted sleep meaning not waking up in the middle of the night two or three times. Children need 8 to 10 hours of sleep each night. There are some people who are able get by with only five or six hours a sleep a night, but this is because they are able to fall asleep fast into deep sleep and are uninterrupted when they sleep. Many of us wake several times during the night thus interrupting the sleeping process and we are then unable to get that uninterrupted sleep we need.

Sleeping too long is also not healthy. You might find that if you sleep longer than you need you will have the same symptoms as if you didn't get enough sleep. You will be tired and feel like you didn't get enough sleep, but do not fall into the trap and attempt to get more sleep, because then you will feel even more tired. This is why many people tend to sleep longer than they need, because they will continue to feel like they need more sleep.

The next element of sleep is the time you go to bed and the time you wake up. It is crucial to retire to bed and wake up the same time every day in order to develop a rhythm or pattern your body can get used to and can count on in order to recover the mind and body. If you are going to bed different times and waking up different times it will throw your body and mind out of balance with your overall health. This can be tough to do since we have work schedules, family events, commitments, and many other things that may require an altering of our schedules. But many of us have control over our sleep schedules yet we choose to watch television, text our friends, or spend the time studying for an exam, doing homework. Many people find themselves staying up late, and then either sleeping late for being sleep deprived hoping to catch up during the weekend, only it doesn't work out that way.

You can notice a huge difference in how you feel and how much energy you have by sticking to a schedule where you are able to go to bed and wake up at the same time every day of the year. You will have to develop a routine that works best with your lifestyle and that of your family. It is hard for those who work odd hours like graveyard or swing shift, but it still can be managed. Do not try to make up the hours of sleep you missed during the week on the weekends or any other time, because it doesn't really work, and it further messes up your sleep schedule. You can take power naps during the day that might help you. But do not nap longer than 15 minutes, or it will cause further problems with your sleep schedule, just like how parents hate it when their child has a late nap or their nap is longer than expected and the child ends up staying up late at night, because they have had too much rest.

It is important to eat a healthy diet, exercise, practice yoga and meditation, and to have your room set up in such a way that it invites a good night's rest. The bed should be comfortable, the room has the ability to get dark even when it is light outside, and it should be able to prevent outside noise. You should not have a television in the room, because it will be too much of a temptation for you to want to watch television at night before bed which for some is a habit to wind down at the end of the day, but even though it might feel like it is winding you down, it is still stimulating the brain making it harder for your brain to be able to process what you have done during the day, making it harder for your to enter into deep REM sleep.

The main function of sleep is to allow the brain time to process all of the information and experiences that took place during the day. This is why it is hard to sleep when the mind is actively trying to go through a lot of information of what happened during the day. This might be that you have a lot of stress you're thinking about, you had a mentally taxing day, or that you are thinking about something coming up in your life. It could also be that you just went through a mentally disturbing or stressful event, such as the death of a loved one, breaking up with someone you love, or getting into a fight with someone.

The first step in falling asleep is being able to slow down the mind and all of the thoughts that are racing through the mind. Even if it is only a single thought it might occupy all of your thoughts and cause you to remain awake because you are thinking about that one thing. This is why it is important to allow your mind to let go of everything before you go to bed. Allow your mind to bring in those thoughts that come across the stage of your mind, and then let them go reserved to come forth in the morning when you are more rested and prepared to thing about them. The worst thing you can do is to attempt to solve the mysteries of the Universe before you go to bed.

Some people like to study and think about things at night when it is quiet, only it is very demanding on the mind and will destroy your sleep and sleep patterns. It is far better to get up early with a good night sleep behind you and you are fresh to think about the problems and things you stressed about the night before. If you get into the pattern of letting go and facing the things you need to do each morning you will be able to get a lot more sleep, and you will do better at solving problems.

Before going to bed say your prayers reflecting on the day making it short, then do breathing meditation. You can then get into a nightly ritual where you meditate, stretch, and get both your mind and body ready for rest. You should avoid eating before bed, watching television, anything that may interfere with allowing your mind to become relaxed. Even strenuous exercise might cause you to remain awake longer because of the added adrenaline into the body. Light exercise like yoga will be more beneficial and allow the mind to relax.

How you wake up may also have a profound impact on your sleep. I do not like the annoying beeping sounds of alarm clocks and watches to be woken up to. I prefer sunrise clocks that simulate the rising of the sun. This is great because there is no annoying beeping, and it helps the body to wake up naturally instead of an alarm. There were times when it felt like my head was hit by a hammer when I woke up with the beeping of an alarm clock, but with the sunrise clock, I feel refreshed and ready to take on the world. The sunrise clocks are more expensive, but well worth every penny spent on them. The sunrise clock does not work if you already get up after the sun goes up, or you are a heavy sleeper and need an anvil to be dropped on your head every morning.

Good sleep will promote healthy bodies and minds. It is important that you sleep well each night. Poor sleeping habits can cause a lot more stress on the body and mind making it difficult to have adequate sleep for a healthy mind and body.

Exercise

"And see that all these things are done in wisdom and order; for it is not requisite that a man should run faster than he has strength. And again, it is expedient that he should win the prize; therefore, all things must be done in order." (Mosiah 4:27)

The scriptures are filled with things we should do, and the prophets are giving us more things we are to do each time at general conference, not to mention our callings in the church, family responsibilities, and attempting to live a good life. Thus the most common excuse not to exercise is, "I am just too busy to exercise, I do not have the time. I really wish I could exercise, I love to ride my bike or weight lift, but when am I going to find the time to do this.

The Lord does not expect you to do more than you are capable of doing, but there is still an element of working hard spiritually, mentally, and physically. It takes a lot of effort to raise a family, fulfill church callings, and work full time to support your family, and then you attempt to squeeze a little personal time in your life, which often means watching television, or something passive. This can just complicate things more in your life, because you will gain weight, not have as much energy as you would like, and your body will start to go through aches and pains form inactivity.

Hard work is an essential part of life. Going to large cities seeing the homeless people, I notice that there is one constant which is lack of activity. I went for a run one morning in Washington DC, and noticed that there were two worlds, those who were not homeless going to work and being active, and those who were homeless and inactive. It was the inactivity of the homeless that bothered me. As I ran through the streets, I felt great getting out and running despite the humidity and the sweat poring down my forehead.

For the first time I truly realized what hell would be like, to spend the rest of eternity not doing anything. It was not my place to judge those who were homeless, but I felt pity for them not because they were homeless, but that they were not active. Many of them had bad health and just sat on benches doing nothing all day except to go to the corner and ask for money so that they could get something to eat. The inactivity of these homeless people not only causes them to have bad physical health but it also affects their spiritual and mental health as well.

I like the analogy of water in a stagnant pond verses a fast flowing river. The water in the pond is disease infested and unhealthy whereas the fast flowing river is healthy because of the flow of the water creating more oxygen in the river and healthy for all of the fish and other animals that rely on the water. Our bodies are the same the more active they are the healthier they are the less active the less healthy they are.

Exercise such as running, swimming, or biking increases the heart rate forcing the heart to pump faster and stronger to get the blood around the body faster. When the blood goes faster around the body it provides the body more importantly the brain with a lot more oxygen and chemicals to allow the body and mind to be healthier. It also has a cleansing affect on the body and mind which results in not getting sick as often and being able to think more clearly. It also gives the body more energy.

Lifting weights, and doing resistant type exercises help to build strength in the muscle skeletal systems of the body. The best treatment for making sure to have strong bones and muscles is to do weight bearing and resistant exercises. Resistant exercises will also help to prevent injuries and improve recovery of injuries.

Stretching and doing yoga will help improve the range of motions in of the muscles. It will help to prevent injury as well, stretching helps to release the stress and tension of the body thus reducing overall stress and helps to improve overall strength and energy. This is one aspect of exercise that is often ignored or overlooked at all of the great benefits that come from stretching.

There are several other key aspects to exercise such as stamina, agility, speed, and overall health that are part of an active lifestyle. In the past my grandparents thought of exercise as taking a walk to the park with the grandchildren, working out in the garden, or doing house work. They never thought of exercise as something separate in their life that they had to do each day in order to be healthy, they thought it was just part of living.

Today exercise is something many people think of as a good thing, only they have no time to do it, and they do not have the energy to exercise after working eight hours behind a desk. There are a lot of fitness enthusiasts who dedicate an hour or two a day to exercise or recreation. You have your joggers and walkers in the morning, your bikers, your sports enthusiasts who play golf, basketball, or soccer religiously. But for many Americans exercise is just an ideal and not a practice.

Many people by the time they are 25 years old have experienced exercise by playing at recess in school, participating in the presidential fitness program, participating in sports in school, on a COMP team, or in the neighborhood. They took one or two classes in high school where they had to run and lift weights. They might have even at one point worked out for a period of time. But they never really got into exercising because they were not interested in it. There are so many more things for them to do, like texting, gaming, and watching television. It is so much more fun to just hang out with friends talking. The idea of setting at least a half an hour a day to exercise never crosses many people's mind, unless it is a temporary fad that they experience in order to lose weight or attempt to get stronger.

Everything about exercise in America is superficial only on the surface with the desire to look better, have more energy, and be healthy, only to do it for a time and then going back to bad habits. Many people do not want to commit to something that requires a lot of effort, a change in lifestyle, and something that requires the rest of their lives to do. Once the workouts become boring and the effort required to keep exercising seems too much people stop exercising.

In order to gain the best benefits from exercise you need to understand some basic fundamentals about exercise. The first is that it requires hard work, hard physical work. This is something many people are unable to do. It all starts with youth, I can immediately tell which children will have a hard time with health in the future, by who complains about it being too hard, too hot, too cold, and they hate sweating. I have taught PE classes where students purposefully sat down and did nothing all period long while the rest of the students played basketball, and they knew that they would fail the class and that the class was a required PE class. They would do nothing and be bored and not graduate from high school, because they did not want to participate in PE.

Not only is exercise hard work, it takes a time commitment. This means at least 30 minutes a day or longer with Sunday as a rest day. You should have at least one day a week when you rest from exercising so that the body can recover and it allows for you to change up your routine and to keep the workouts interesting. The commitment also extends to exercising on a regular basis for the rest of your life. It needs to be part of your daily routine just as important as brushing your teeth, using the restroom, and saying your prayers.

The hardest part of exercise is getting started and sticking with it. There are a lot of fitness programs out there ranging from intense workouts for advanced athletes and less intense workouts for novices. There are martial arts workouts, yoga workouts, weight lifting workouts, and then there are the exercise machines with their own workouts. Do not get sucked into buying something you will never use, do your research and look into what might work best for you.

The best approach to developing an exercise routine is to look at what you want to accomplish, your fitness goals, and how it will fit into your life. You can try out and look at other workouts, but until you make it your own you will not make it apart of your life. This is the major reason why fad routines, and exercise machines come and go. Do not rely on other people's success stories either, you need to have your own success stories. Just read the fine print which states that results will vary. The truth is that the results you get will be different from other people's because your body, mind, and life is different from other people's lives.

The key things you need to include in your workout would be to have endurance exercises such as jogging, swimming, biking, walking, and hiking. Anything you can do for a sustained period of time and builds endurance and focus on the heart and lungs this is why these exercises are known as cardiovascular exercise. Another name is aerobic exercises because you are able to do these exercises with sustained air or oxygen without getting out of breathe fast as in anaerobic exercise like weight lifting. I choose to call these exercises endurance exercises because the help with endurance. Since these exercise work on endurance and help with the heart and lungs they are the most important and should be done on a daily basis with at least one rest day during the week. You can choose to do these three times a week for twenty minutes which is the minimum recommended by experts, but I prefer to do them on a daily basis changing up with jogging, biking, hiking, and swimming, sometimes doing one, sometimes doing all of them in the summer to increase my overall health and endurance.

You should also include strength or resistance exercises that helps to improve strength. These exercises would include weight lifting, resistant bands, and weight bearing exercises such as push-ups and pull-ups. Because these exercises often tears down the muscle you will experience being sore. It is important to allow the muscles to recover from being sore which means at least a day's rest before exercising again. This means that you might weight lift for three days a week with one rest day in-between each. You should include all of the major muscle groups such as the shoulders, arms, chest, back, abs, quadriceps, and calves. Just remember when you are exercising you need to shoot for an overall workout, one in which you will work out all of the muscles in the body and not just one group creating an unhealthy imbalance in the body.

The last form of exercise would be that of stretching which I call flexibility exercises because they increase the range of motion or flexibility in a person's body. These are done doing one of three types of stretches; the static stretch is a stretch that is held for a period of time, the ballistic stretch which is where bouncing is taken place to force the stretch which is not recommended because it can cause injury, and finally the dynamic stretching where there is movement that is involved in the stretching. Both static and dynamic stretches has their uses and benefits in your workout. Dynamic stretching will help to increase your flexibility faster than the other stretching and is used in martial arts, yoga, and ballet to improve flexibility.

Once you have included endurance, strength, and flexibility exercise in your routine you will need to come up with a format of your routine. It is good to start out simple and slow and then make it harder and longer to improve the intensity of the workout and improve your overall health. The main thing to remember when doing any workout would be to be focused on the workout at all times. The only times I have gotten hurt while working out was when I was not focused on what I was doing. The workout goes smoothly and does not take as much time when you are focused to the point you are concentrating on every move. If you perform a move incorrect or an exercise that is done wrong you can injure yourself and you will not gain the most from your workout.

If you are doing dumbbell curls in order to get bigger stronger arms, and you use too much of your back, you will be making your back muscles stronger while avoiding the biceps. Concentrate on every exercise and make sure you are doing it correctly. It doesn't matter how much you can lift, or being able to impress others. It matters about doing the exercise right in order to do what it was intended to do.

The correct procedure of a workout should be to first participate in warming up your muscles which could be a walk, a short jog, jumping rope, or doing something a little less aggressive such as Tai Chi Chuan. This allows the muscles to warm up and the blood to flow throughout the body. With the muscles warmed up then you will be able to stretch or do some yoga. Then you can do an endurance exercise like running and this should be done for at least twenty minutes. You then can go into weight lifting or resistance exercises. You should include all of the muscles, do at least three sets of each with at least 12 reps.

The best way to do the resistant exercises is to superset or do circuit training where you go from one exercise to the next without resting. You could go from bench pressing to doing arm curls, or leg presses. This is the fastest and most efficient way to workout, and you help to increase the blood flow in the body. It is important to continue to stretch and massage the muscles in order to keep them loose and ready for the rest of the workout.

At the end of the workout you need to do a cool down which is similar to the warm up except that you are attempting to cool down the body which allows the bodies muscles to work better and you have a better recovery rate from one workout to the next. The cool down can include massage which is important in muscle health and it also helps with relieving stress might also include some form of meditation as well.

Consistency is the key to success when it comes to exercise. You need to be consistent on working out on a regular basis in order for you to see results. It might take several weeks before you see a change in your life and are able to feel better, have more energy, and be able to do things that you never thought you could do before. You will need to increase the intensity of the workout from time to time in order to get stronger, and not get bored with the workouts. Do not give up, because your life or in other words your health depends on it!

Nutrition

"And again, verily I say unto you, all wholesome herbs God hath ordained for the constitution, nature, and use of man." (D&C 89:10)

Section 89 of the Doctrine and Covenants mainly focuses on diet when it comes to health. It gives several key elements that are critical in today's health. The first it talks about the last days and how there will be those who will attempt to do things to deceive people. We see this in advertisements for alcohol, the new products with energy and sport drinks, we also see this in people who would want to legalize illegal drugs in an attempt to stop the drug wars that is costing the country millions of dollars and thousands of people have died in other countries over it. But the answer isn't in legalization of illegal substances, or in a futile war against drug cartels the answer comes through the Word of Wisdom which is outlined in section 89. If everyone would just follow the principles outlined in section 89 and the counsel of the living prophets then these problems would be solved as well as the destructive forces of cancer, heart disease, cancer, and many other ailments caused by poor diet.

Section 89 continues in verses five through seven to talk about how alcohol is not for the belly, or should not be taken into the body. Alcoholic beverages alone accounts for billions of dollars in medical expenses, domestic violence, automobile accidents, and several other alcohol related actions. The impact of alcohol in the world today cannot fully be realized because of the impact it has on families, especially children through domestic violence which results in abuse neglect, and abandonment. There are also children who were born with fetal alcohol syndrome who have a hard time functioning in society. The best defense against this is to simply teach not to drink alcoholic beverages. There are some studies that suggest having some alcohol in your diet is healthy, but these studies are not 100 percent accurate and the risks of the effects of alcohol far out way any benefits.

Tobacco use is talked about in verse 8. Research proves that tobacco use alone kills an average of over 400,000 people a year in the United States. Just think of how many people this adds up to over the years. More people have died from tobacco use than all of the wars, diseases, and natural disasters combined. It is simple do not use tobacco. It isn't the death that is the worst part of it, it is how the people die that is the story. Tobacco kills slowly, a person is eaten up by cancer, or slowly suffocates to death through lung cancer, or emphysema. If you observe people who are addicted to smoking it is not a fun habit. I personally would not want to wake up for the rest of my life with a migraine headache and cough up a lung every morning.

Verse 9 talks about hot drinks which the prophets have told us means coffee and tea, both of which have a lot of caffeine in them. Caffeine has been linked to several side effects as well as low birth weight, premature children, and miscarriages. It can be just as destructive as nicotine when it comes to being a stimulant increasing heart rate and putting stress on the body. People can have sever withdrawals when they attempt to stop. Caffeinated soft drinks can be just as bad along with energy drinks, because they contain not only caffeine but a lot of refined sugar which can further increase the heart rate as well as the sugar level in the blood stream all of which puts a lot of stress on the body. It is important to avoid all drinks that contain caffeine in them. They are especially not good for children.

When it comes to hot chocolate, and herbal teas, chocolate contains some caffeine, but not enough to cause to much alarm, and dark chocolate has some health benefits with its antioxidants, and many herbal teas are beneficial. Be careful not to have the drinks too hot, for obvious reasons the heat will burn the mouth and throat. Herbs are spoken of in verses 10 and 11. In China herbs have been used for medicine long before the west came up with drugs to use to combat illness. Herbs that are used with skill can do wonders. You need to do a lot of research and make sure that you are using the herb properly or you may experience unhealthy side effects.

In verses 12 and 13 it talks about eating meat. It talks about eating meat on a regular basis and not just in times of famine or during the winter. The passage also talks of using meat sparingly. In the past meat was a main staple in the winter time because of the scarcity of grains, fruits, and vegetables. Lewis and Clark on their two year expedition lived mostly on meat from hunting and fishing. Since we have readily access to a lot of different choices of food to eat, we do not have to eat as much meat even in the winter time and during times of famine.

"And whoso forbiddeth to abstain from meats, that man should not eat the same is not ordained of God; For, behold, the beasts of the field and the fowls of the air, and that which cometh of the earth, is ordained for the use of man for food and for raiment, and that he might have in

111

abundance. And wo be unto man that sheddeth blood or that wasteth flesh and hath no need." (D&C 49:18,19,21)

The Lord says that it is not good for someone to be a vegetarian or tell someone to be a vegetarian. People who are strictly Vegan vegetarians are not as healthy as those who eat meat properly. They lack a lot of the essential amino acids their bodies need. But verse 21 also talks about how it is important not to kill for sport and waste the meat, and to have respect for the animals. We have gotten to the point where we waste a lot of meat and take the meat we buy in the grocery store or in a restaurant for granted. This can be a very bad think and many of us are suffering from it because of all of the manipulation and hormones that are given to livestock. There are many more people who suffer from allergies and other ailments because of the genetic manipulation of farmers and ranchers.

In section 89 verse 14 through 17 talks about the use of grains, fruits and vegetables that are good for us with an emphasis on wheat for man. Wheat is a grain that can last for several years in food storage and can be used for breads, cereals, and pastas. The whole wheat is the best. The white flour often used in a variety of pastries and baking is void of the fiber and nutrients that makes wheat healthy. Many people are now becoming allergic to wheat and wheat products with the gluten, primarily because of how food is processed these days causing the body to reject such foods. People have to seek out other sources of grains besides wheat, because of their body's rejection of it.

When it comes to diet and nutrition there is a couple of simple things to remember. There are six nutrients the body needs three do not have calories and three that do have calories. We need these six nutrients in order to survive. There are vitamins, minerals, and water all of which do not have calories, but are essential in order to survive and live healthy. These nutrients are found in the foods we eat, and some people take them in the form of pills and bottled water. As for vitamins and minerals the best source is natural from our foods, it can be harmful to consumer too many vitamins and minerals and can even reach toxic levels if you are not careful. Taking too many vitamins and minerals will only hurt your health, so be careful what you take. As for water just make sure that the water is clean without contaminants which can be done through filtering the water, there are a lot of great filters out there and there is also UV lights that are effective in killing germs. It is recommended to have eight glasses of water a day, but I find this to be too much water for me. I believe that you can find the right amount of water you consume each day, just make sure to have at least a few glasses of pure clean water a day and not substitute it with fruit juice, soda pop, or other drinks.

The next three nutrients are; fats, carbohydrates, and protein. The problem most people face is having the right combination of the three in their diet. Having too much of any one nutrient is not good, and having too little is not good either. Fat contains the most calories with 10 calories per gram for fats. Our bodies need essential oils or fats in order to perform its proper functions like transport things around in the blood system. But we do not need a lot of fat in our diet around 10% of our diet should come through fat.

Protein is also essential to help our bodies work properly such as repairing and building muscle. Like fats we do not need too much protein for our bodies. It is important to eat a variety of protein sources such as dairy products, fish, poultry, cattle, bean, and nuts. 15% of your diet should come from protein. Attempt to eat lean meat, and avoid as much cholesterol as you can.

Carbohydrates should make up 75% of your diet because they contain the vitamins, minerals, and calories necessary to get you through the day. There are two types of Carbohydrates the simple and complex. Simple refers to the refined sugars. They burn fast and will give the body a spike of sugar for a short period of time and then there will be a crash. This is why simple sugars are often referred to as having empty calories. After eating a candy bar you will not feel full and even might feel empty and thus craving some more candy bars or anything else that comes to mind or is readily available. This is the number one cause of obesity in people today. The empty calories cause people to eat more food than their bodies can't handle and it is stored as fat.

Complex calories are what you need to focus on in your diet. These are whole grains, fruits and vegetables that are dense in nutrients. This means eating whole grain wheat, brown and wild rice, and eating salad with cucumbers, spinach, carrots, peas, and a variety of other vegetables. Fruit has antioxidants that will help to combat cellular degeneration. The berries are rich in vitamins and minerals as well as antioxidants. blueberries, strawberries, blackberries, and grapes are all up to the challenge to help improve your health.

Fruits, vegetables, and grains also contain fiber which is essential in dietary track it helps to control the flow of food through the digestive system. It cleans the digestive system and helps to prevent digestive illnesses. Just like with all other things it is important not to take too much or you will have problems, and if you are not used to having a lot of fiber in your diet it will take some time to get used to.

Calories are important to keep track in your diet. They help to provide energy for the body and help the body to keep going. The brain as well as the rest of the body needs calories to provide enough energy to function normally. In the United States we tend to have too much calories, which results in gaining weight and becoming unhealthy. Restaurants serve us with too many calories for the meal we are eating. On average most people do not need to eat more than 2,000 calories a day, and most nutritional labels are based on a 2,000 calorie diet. It is easy to consume a lot of calories especially since a lot of foods now contain more calories. Drinks can be a major contributor to consuming too many calories.

Many soft drinks contain more than 170 calories per serving, and many people will consume three or four soft drinks a day which adds up to over 500 empty calories with no nutrients other than simple sugars. This means that one fourth of the calorie intake comes from empty calories that do little in the way of helping our health. A fast food meal can easily contain more than a thousand calories and this is for one meal. A lot of those calories are from empty calories as well which causes you to be hungry only a few hours after consuming those thousand calories. You can easily reach the two thousand calories and even up to three or more thousand calories before the day is up. What the body cannot use it will get ride off in waste or store it as fat.

The simple formula is to consume only the calories you will use. If you eat more calories than your body will use you will gain weight. If you eat less calories than your body uses then you will lose weight. It takes a while for you to determine how many calories your body uses, especially when you add exercise into the picture. But if you are eating only an extra five hundred calories a day you can gain up to four pounds a month. Five hundred calories adds up to a cheese burger, or a large order of fries, or a 36 ounce soft drink.

In order to have a healthy diet, you simply have to eat a lot of nutrient dense foods such as whole grains, fruits, and vegetables. Watch how much sweets, fats, and proteins you eat, and make sure you are not eating a lot of unnecessary calories. I would avoid drinking too much soda pop, eating foods with refined sugars, high fructose corn syrup, and foods with a lot of cholesterol.

Some other healthy habits would be not to eat two hours before going to bed. Do not eat in front of the television. Eat small meals throughout the day and large meals. Chose healthy meals while eating out and sharing meals with members of the family it will save you a lot of money and a lot of hours in the gym to work off the extra weight. If you have a lot of leftovers at the restaurant then you ordered too much food. If you leave the restaurant stuffed and very full, you ordered too much food as well. Make a habit of fixing healthy meals at home and eating together as a family.

Get into planning food storage and fixing meals from your food storage so that you can rotate the food storage and get used to meals you can make from your food storage. Come up with inventive ways to cook meals on a grill, or a camp stove. Get used to fixing meals from scratch and planning out your own garden.

It is important to be able to get closer to the foods we eat. The more distant and impersonal the food we eat the less healthy the food is. Attempt to get the freshest fruits and vegetables you can buy. Try to buy organic foods that do not contain any chemicals, or additives that may be harmful to your health.

Making a habit of saying a blessing on the food you eat, and having a spirit of gratitude is also an essential element of your diet and will help to connect the spiritual aspect of our diets with the spirit. The more we pay attention to our spirits, and bodies the more we will be able to eat better and as we listen to our spirits we will know which foods are healthy and which are not and have the willpower to eat a healthy diet and not eat more calories than we need for the day.

Fasting once a month is also an essential part of your diet. It helps to cleanse the body from toxins and it also humbles us to the fact that we are so blessed with the abundance of the food we have. If we use food the way it is intended it will bring us joy, long life, and wisdom. All of which is given to us as a blessing for following the commandments in the scriptures.

"Verily, this is fasting and prayer, or in other words, rejoicing and prayer. And insamuch as ye do these things with thanksgiving, with cheerful hearts, and countenances, not with much laughter, for this is sin, but with a glad heart and a cheerful countenance. Verily I say, that inasmuch as ye do this, the fullness of the earth is yours, the beasts of the field and the fowls of the air, and that which climbeth upon the trees and walketh upon the earth; Yea, and the herb, and the good things which come of the earth, whether for food or for rainment, or for houses, or for barns, or for orchards, or for gardens, or for vineyards; Yea, all things which come of the earth, in the season thereof, are made for the benefit and the use of man, both to please the eye and to gladden the heart." (D&C 59:14 – 18)

Hygiene

Hygiene is a big part of health that is often overlooked, because we normally already develop hygiene habits during our youth. We brush our teeth morning and night, take a shower every day, and wash our hands before we eat. Yet in the same manner of hygiene we might not keep our homes as clean, or do not take care of our outer bodies as much as we should. It is important to keep our feet dry, clean, and the nails cut on a regular basis. We need to wash our bodies frequently, brush our teeth, floss our teeth, and use sunscreen when we go outside and are exposed to the sun.

It is important to protect our eyes by wearing polarized sun glasses when going outside, and to dress according to the weather. You can use eye drops and keep your eyes clean. Do not listen to loud music or noises that may damage the ear. The damage to the hearing could be made permanent. Those working in jobs that are exposed to loud noise need to wear ear plugs and many need to wear eye protective goggles.

It is important to always think of safety while at work and home. It only takes a moment of carelessness to destroy a person's life. I would recommend becoming familiar with your companies emergency plan, and to have one at your home. You should become first-aid, CPR certified so that you would be able to act in the case of an emergency.

To Do List

1. Wake up and go to bed at the same time every day.
2. Develop a bedtime routine and stick with it.
3. Develop a personalized routine that includes endurance, flexibility, and strength exercises as well as including a warm-up and cool-down in your workout.
4. Eat a well balanced diet with nutrient dense foods such as fruits, vegetables, and whole grains.
5. Obey the Word of Wisdom by not consuming anything that will harm your body.
6. Fast once a month, bless your food at each meal and give thanks for all that you have.
7. Start a healthy garden with vegetables you will eat, and plant fruit bushes and trees.
8. Maintain a healthy supply of food storage that you use on a regular basis to be able to come up with meals you and your family will eat.
9. Watch your calories and do not eat too much during the day. Eat small meals of no more than 400 calories per meal.
10. Keep yourself clean by taking a shower daily, brushing and flossing twice a day, and keeping yourself well groomed.

Chapter Six: Relationships or Social Health

"A new commandment I give unto you, that ye love one another; as I have loved you, that ye also love one another." (ST John 13:34)

Social health can be the most complicated when it comes to overall health. We are social creatures and need to love, and be loved in order to be healthy. Those whose social health suffers their physical, mental, and spiritual health suffers as well. Social health can be very complicated because it involves, family, friends, co-workers, and classmates as well as neighbors and strangers we encounter. People whose mental, spiritual, or physical health that is not functioning can cause problems with their social health as well.

Communication

There are many aspects to social health with the most important one being communication. The first step to being an effective communicator is to be able to listen. This comes from being an active listener. Many people fall into the trap of being a passive listener or a selective listener only listening to the things that are important to us. But when someone is saying something it is important to them, and in order for us to be able to connect with that person we need to make what they are telling us important to us as well. By being an active listener and making what we are listening to important to us, we can get to know the person a lot better and be able to empathize with them better and understand where they are coming from and what they are attempting to tell us.

Think about when you are excited about tell something to someone and they seem less excited how you feel, or think about how you feel when you tell something to someone and they are excited about what you are telling them. This is what happens when you listen to others as well. Being an active listener is also asking people to clarify what they told you, or expanding on what they are talking about. You might also say something like, "So you are telling me this," or "Let me see if I understood you. You are saying this."

Being an active listener also means to be able to follow through with what you are listening to. If someone tells you about how they are going through a hard time, then the next time you see them tell them how you are concerned with them and you were thinking about them. This will not only make them feel better that you remembered them, it will help you to be able to understand people better and connect with them on a more personal level.

Once you have mastered the art of listening you will then be able to communicate with people better. The next part of communication is to be able to convey your thoughts, feelings, and ideas to others. This can be hard for people because of the fear of how they feel the other person will react to what they express. It can be further complicated when you express your feelings to someone and their reaction to what you said is not what you expected or turns out bad. It is hard to tell what any person might say or do when you tell them something. You might be genuine in expressing your feelings in a positive manner, and the person you are talking with might explode in anger not from what you said, but because he is having a bad day and what you said triggered something inside.

It is important to be enthusiastic about things you are excited about, honest and genuine about everything you say, and mindful of the other person's feelings, ideas, and thoughts. If you are less genuine and are selfish in your manner of speaking then the person you are speaking to will pick up on this and will not respond in a favorable manner. Do not try to push an agenda on someone who is unwilling to listen to it or has their own agenda. It is very hard to convince someone when no one is willing to bend a little. Honest sincere gratitude and praise can go a long way in setting at ease the conversation and will help you to be able to communicate with the other person better.

When you are talking with another person pay attention to all of the non-verbal cues they are giving. If a person is backing away from you, she is telling you that they are attempting to end the conversation. It might mean that she doesn't want to talk with you, or it might mean that she just has an appointment she needs to get to. If you sense that the person wants to end the conversation do not attempt to continue to talk with the person, because that person will then start to resent the time she is spending with you. It is important to honor the wishes of the person you are talking with even if it is just non-verbal.

You can also notice the eyes. If the person is having strong eye contact with you it might mean that he is interested in what you are talking, or it might mean that he is upset with you and is starting to be confrontational. If he has poor eye contact and does not look at you it might mean that he is shy and doesn't know what to say, or it might mean that he is not interested in the conversation and is attempting to end the conversation.

Some non-verbal signals are obvious others are not. It is important to be able to read them so that you are able to understand what the other person might be thinking or feeling. Practice paying attention to non-verbal body language. You might need to watch television without the sound to see the non-verbal cues the characters have when they are talking with others actors. They will often over exaggerate their body language in order to convey their thoughts and feelings to the audience.

You might even want to practice body language of your own so that you can be a more interesting speaker.

People like to listen to people who are animated and use body language to tell part of the story. Two speakers can give the same speech, one very animated and the other without any non-verbal cues. The one that is animated will be better received by the audience than the one who is not.

Communication is not about you, it is about the other person you are communicating with. Make sure you get to know the person you are talking with in order to be able to break through to them. If you do not know them, you will miss a lot of opportunities that could change your life. When two people are able to talk with each other as active listeners and paying attention to their body language, being genuine and engaged in understanding what the other person is saying there become a chemistry that will bring them closer together.

Conflict Resolution

Conflict in a relationship is inevitable. It seems like the closer you are to a person there is more potential for conflict. By nature humans are social creatures and with the social comes the conflict with others in order to compete with others we need to attempt to persuade others that our way is better than their way, or that their way is not worth doing.

Through history conflict was resolved by mediation, arbitration, or by the courts. The main focus of the conflict resolution is compromise where both parties agree upon something that they are willing to give up. This can help in the short term, but it can also create further problems in the future. Whenever someone has to give up something that they hold dear to their hearts it means that they will hold that against the person and the conflict is still present only suppressed for the time being to surface later.

The civil war was the result of decades of compromise over slavery. There are some things that take more drastic measures to solve. But it may be simply to come together with the person you are have a problem with and to talk it out resolving the conflict through compassion and understanding. Try to use Christ as the example where he was patient and attempted to resolve conflicts through explaining the situation. Like the woman who was taken into adultery the men asked Christ what to do, he drew in the sand for a moment for the men to think about what they were asking then he told them that if any of them were without sin they should caste the first stone at the woman. The men left and Christ told the woman to leave and sin no more without any bloodshed occurring. Later the Savior answered questions with a question when asked about what should be lawful on the Sabbath. They were trying to condemn him from helping people on the Sabbath and he asked them if they had helped their animals on the Sabbath which many of them had, and asked helping their animals was more important than helping people on the Sabbath.

There were times when Jesus had to deal with people in a different way such as the money changers in the temple. He did not chase them off with a whip and overturn the tables out of anger, but did it to make a point that the temple was a sacred place and they made it out to be place where the people were trying get rich. Later Jesus refused to talk with King Harod because he knew that he could not say a word to the wicked man that was of any benefit. Harod was the instrument of killing John the Baptist Jesus' cousin and friend.

So when it comes to conflict resolution there might be a time when you just have to remain silent, and a time when you overturn tables. But most of the time you should be able to just talk with someone about the conflict, if this doesn't work you might need to get a natural third party to help mediate the conflict. It is important to attempt to come to a win win situation where everyone involved in the conflict leaves feeling happy and not disappointed about the outcome. If you can leave as friends it is so much better than to leave feeling like nothing was resolved and there will be complications further down the road.

The conflict in Israel is a perfect example of what not to do in conflict resolution. All of the people involved simply want to be able to live in peace only they want power in the government. Their idea is that they want lasting peace for their people, and they do not trust the others to make sure that will happen. No one is willing to forgive the other and move forward in a cooperation effort to make Israel a strong country with a lot of economic potential. Instead of helping each other they are fighting each other. All of the people in Israel could have a wonderful life, if they were to just give up on seeking revenge for what has happened in the past. Instead of looking at what they can accomplish they are looking at what they can do to blame the others for.

Leadership

"If your actions inspire others to dream more, learn more, do more, and become more, you area a leader." John Quincy Adams

Leadership is more complex than simply communicating with others, being a good listener and practicing conflict resolution. It is a matter of working with others and inspiring others to do their best. You might say that you do not have to worry about being a leader, and that you are better as a follower than a leader. But all of us at one point in our life will be given the chance to be a leader, all of us will be placed in that role if only for a moment, and it is at that time when our true character will come out, and it will be important that we are prepared for when that time comes.

We might become a leader to our younger brothers, or sisters. It might be that we are placed in charge of others in the role of being a beehive president, deacon's quorum president, or patrol leader in scouts. There is no surprise that the church offers so many leadership roles and opportunities as well as social activities. It is an essential part of life. Not only will you have the opportunity to be placed in a leadership role in church, but you will have that opportunity at home with your family especially when you become a parent which is the ultimate leadership role, then comes times when you will have leadership roles at work and in the community. There is only one president of the United States of America at any given time and the chances that you will be president is very slim, but being president is not as important a role as serving as relief society president, or elder's quorum president, or being a good father or mother.

Many of the leadership roles you will have in your life will be minor ones in which you will be in charge of a handful of people. But you will have the opportunity to have a huge impact on those people on that will last a lifetime and may influence them to take a path in life, or be able to help teach them a valuable skill. So when it comes to leadership everyone should take notes in what it takes to be a good leader.

Let's first look at what is a bad leader.

"Behold, there are many called, but few are chosen. And why are they not chosen? Because their hearts are set so much upon the things of this world, and aspire to the honors of men, that they do not learn this one lesson- That the rights of the priesthood are inseparably connected with the powers of heaven, and that the power of heaven cannot be controlled nor handled only upon the principles of righteousness. That may be conferred upon us, it is true; but when we undertake to cover our sins, or to gratify our pride, our vain ambitions, or to exercise control or dominion or compulsion upon the souls of the children of men, in any degree of unrighteousness, behold the heavens withdraw themselves; the Spirit of the Lord is grieved; and when it is withdrawn, Amen to the priesthood or the authority of that man." (D&C 121:34-37)

A bad leader is one who is in it for himself he is selfish and prideful. He will use his power and authority to gratify his own will and desires and hurt others in the process. Leaders who abuse those they lead are not good leaders, and will only lead into rebellion and conflict between the leader and those he leads. This has been seen throughout history with all of the leaders of the past. Those who lead for their own purpose fell hard without the support of their followers while those who were great leaders were the ones who commanded the respect of those in whom he lead.

If we take a look at the same section in the Doctrine and Covenants which is about the priesthood which is the governing power and authority of the leaders of the church it talks about the proper way to lead.

"No power or influence can or ought to be maintained by virtue of the priesthood, only by persuasion, by long-suffering, by gentleness and meekness, and by love unfeigned; By kindness, and pure knowledge, which shall greatly enlarge the soul without hypocrisy, and without guile- Reproving betimes with sharpness, when moved upon by the Holy Ghost; and then showing forth afterwards an increase of love toward him whom thou hast reproved, lest he esteem thee to be his enemy;" (D&C 121:41-43)

It is important that as a leader you show kindness and gentleness to those you lead, convey knowledge to those you lead without being a hypocrite, and correcting those you lead when the Holy Ghost moves you to do so and afterwards showing love towards the person. The key is to be guided by the Spirit when you lead and to use this to help those you lead. You will be given the authority and the blessings to lead those you are given to be in charge of.

A leader needs to have humility where she is willing to admit when she is wrong, willing to accept help from others, and have a willingness to continue to learn from others. As a leader you will often learn far more from those you lead than they will learn from you and the experience you have as a leader will give you a lot of wisdom that will help you further down in your life. Humility is the key to openness, tolerance, and the ability to gain trust and respect to those you are in charge of.

Leaders need integrity in order to build the trust and the loyalty that is necessary to be able to lead. If those you are in charge of do not trust or respect you they will not be willing to do things for you. In the end you should be able to be strong enough through your integrity to be able to be the iron rode in which people hold on to in order to get through the mist of darkness in life. You should be getting your strength and integrity through Christ and be guided by the Holy Ghost in your efforts to perform your duties as a leader. Integrity means doing what you say you will do and not giving promises you cannot keep. It means doing your job no matter what it takes and fulfilling your bargain with others even if it means self sacrifice.

Courage is often associated with leadership, it is an often misunderstood character trait. Some might say that courage is when someone runs into a burning building to save someone, or lead a charge up a hill with the enemy shooting at them. But courage could be as simple as taking on the responsibility of being a parent and being there for her children. It could be having the courage to stand and give a two minute talk in church about the atonement. It could be standing up for someone else who is being bullied. Courage could be the willingness to go home teaching or visiting teaching. Courage is standing up and taking charge when no one else will take on the responsibility. Courage is standing up for your beliefs and taking a side that is not popular with others. It is through this courage that leaders are about to shine and help others to have the same courage.

The greatest courage is to be able to rise above challenges and trials in your life and to continue forward doing your best. When Theodore Roosevelt was a child he was ill most of the time. He could have given up hope of ever playing like the other children and having a normal life, but he with the encouragement of his father exercised and gained strength in his body to be able to go forward in life. When his mother and wife died on the same day he also could have given up and had a quiet life, but he moved forward. He could have sat around as Assistant Secretary of the Navy while men when off to fight in Cuba during the Spanish American War, but he put together his own special unit and went off to war leading his men up San Juan Hill. Roosevelt could have came back home and retired, but he went on to be vice president and then president of the United States.

As president of the United States he boldly went about securing the wilderness and forest areas of the United States and went up against big business as well as many other issues that were not popular for him to touch at the time. When he left being a president he went off to travel in Africa and the Amazon. He came back disappointed at how Taft was running the country and decided to run against him creating his own party. When he was shot by an assassin before giving a speech he went ahead and gave the speech despite having had been shot only moments before. His family embodied his courageous spirit with his sons going off to fight in World War I. Roosevelt himself an old man attempted to get back into the fight during the war and died later in 1919 at age 60 from a heart attack. Later one of his sons fought in World War II receiving the Medal of Honor.

Roosevelt with his efforts was involved in several things including promoting the scouting organization which was newly established in the United States, conserving millions of acres of land to be preserved for future generations, and many more things that showed his quality of being an effective leader.

"I wish to preach, not the doctrine of ignoble ease, but the doctrine of the strenuous life, the life of toil and effort of labor and strife; to preach that highest form of success which comes, not to the man who desires mere easy peace, but to the man who does not shrink from danger, from hardship, or from bitter toil, and who out of these wins the splendid ultimate triumph." Theodore Roosevelt, Chicago, Illinois speech April 10, 1899.

Other examples of true leaders might be seen in the presidents of the church and the modern prophets. Joseph Smith despite being poor and having gone through a lot of trials as a boy took on the responsibility of securing the golden plates and translating the Book of Mormon, and later organizing the church. At any point in his life he could have given it up and lived a peaceful life as a farmer, but he took up the charge and went about preaching the gospel and organizing the church into what we have today. He never once attempted to get gain, or become higher than anyone else in the church. He showed his humanity and humbleness by playing with the children and leading by example.

Joseph Smith lead the saints through the challenges they faced in Ohio, Missouri, and Illinois. He was able to keep the church together long enough for it to have a solid foundation with the twelve apostles and Brigham Young to lead the church when he died. Many of the leaders of the church in the early days were truly great leaders. Brigham Young lead the saints to the west where they established a settlement that would have rivaled many countries at the time. The Utah Territory was a place where the people were self sufficient and didn't need to rely upon outside influences.

You do not have to compare yourself with other leaders, you just have to develop the discipline it takes to be a leader remembering to be humble, courageous, and have integrity in all that you do. The discipline involved in becoming a great leader means keeping your body, mind, and spirit healthy through exercise, diet, reading a lot of books, and keeping the church part of your life fulfilling all of the responsibilities of being a parent, spouse, and church leader. It means working long hours to improve on your leadership skills and abilities. It means building strong relationships with others.

Family

"The Family is ordained of God." The Family: a proclamation to the world, Gordon B. Hinkley September 23, 1995 General Relief Society Meeting.

When the Proclamation of the Family first came out it was widely used and accepted by members of the church and praised by many other people worldwide. Since then it has been read and used by just about all of the members of the church. It is an extremely important statement about family and outlines what families are and what makes up healthy families. Let's take a look at the Lord's view of family and compare it to the world's view.

The first thing is marriage. The world looks as marriage as just a ceremony often times an elaborate celebration in which families spend a lot of money to make an impression on others. Marriage is often cheapened with divorce rates high in both the United States and Canada, and many people believing that there is no real commitment in a marriage and a couple can get divorces easily. There are many couples who choose not to get married and live together instead with no commitment at all. Then there is the campaign to allow same sex marriages which changes the balance of a marriage which is between a man and a woman.

By nature with Ying and Yang from the beginning of time there are opposites and there is the man and the woman. There is no marriage without this. A same sex marriage is going against nature, against God, and against the heart and soul of families.

The Lord's way is, "Marriage between man and woman is essential to His eternal plan, children are entitled to birth within the bonds of matrimony, and to be reared by a father and a mother who honor martial vows with complete fidelity." (The Family a proclamation to the world)

The Plan of Salvation or of Happiness cannot be fulfilled without marriage between a woman and a man, preferably righteous couples who are married in the temple and who are devoted to each other and are able to be eternal companions. Children deserve to have two parents who can teach and guide them throughout their lives. Many children suffer because they only have one parent, or are born out of the bonds of matrimony. Children who only have one parent are less likely to get an education, get a good job, and get into a positive relationship. The cycle of poverty continues with the next generation when there is only one parent. There are many success stories of single parents raising successful children, but this is only because the parent is strong and righteous teaching her children through example and discipline.

The family in the world not only is made up of single parents, it is also made up of step parents, boyfriends, girlfriends, grandparents raising their grandchildren, parents who are drug abusers, criminals, and very dysfunctional families were there are several abuses going on in the family. There are many abuses that are often overlooked or ignored by society which can be very damaging to the children such as parents who work and leave their children home alone for long periods of time without supervision. Parents who are extremely verbally abusive to children and their spouse using swear words on a regular basis, and demeaning them daily for not living up to their expectations. There are parents who expose their children to second hand smoke, get their children addicted to caffeine, and habits of over eating and laziness.

The family creates the foundation for overall health of a child. Many children spend the first twenty plus years in the home, and if it is an abusive home or one that has taught poor health habits those habits and the results of the abuse last a lifetime. This is why there is a cycle of abuse, obesity, and poor health among the lower classes and even middle and high classes of society that last several generations until there is a break in habits, traditions, and ideas. The same holds true for families who pride themselves in establishing healthy habits. This is why many of the great musicians come from families who are musical, the great athletes come from families who are athletic, the education families come from families that are athletic. Many of the children follow the same footsteps as their parents because it is what they are familiar with and it is what they tend to be good at because they have seem examples of it as well.

"Happiness in family life is most likely to be achieved when founded upon the teachings of the Lord Jesus Christ. Successful marriages and families are established and maintained on principles of faith, prayer, repentance, forgiveness, respect, love, compassion, work, and wholesome recreational activities." (The Family; a proclamation to the world)

It is important to follow the teachings of Christ through his modern prophets and to keep in mind these in marriage and in the family. It is through the teachings of

Christ that true happiness comes in families. The Family is the only way to pure happiness as it is in the Plan of Salvation. The biggest concept of the church is eternal families. In order to build eternal families we need to have it while on the earth. If you do not have an eternal family on filled with happiness on this earth you will not have it in the next.

It is important to build faith and trust in the family with parents doing what they say they will do. Children pick up on this really quick if a parent promises something, but then later changes his mind. Family members must have faith in each other to be able to rely on each other and help each other when there is a crisis situation. If you cannot have faith in your family then who can you have faith in. This is why those who do not have anyone in the family to have faith in has lost their faith and hope in life and become hopeless to the things in life.

Prayer is essential in the family. Family prayer can be done in the morning, at night, and during meals. It should also be done before traveling anywhere and doing family activities. Prayer invites the Lord in as a member of the family and ensures the guidance of the Holy Ghost when the family is attempting to make an important decision. It is one essential ingredient in building testimonies of the gospel in the family.

Families need to have repentance and forgiveness as part of the makeup of the family. With a willingness to forgive family members knowing that they will make mistakes and will make wrong decisions form time to time. Along with this it is important to be humble repent of things you have done to other members of your family swallowing your pride and ask for forgiveness. It is the parable of the prodigal son that embodies this. If a child strays from the right things in life, it is the nature of a parent to be able to be there for them when they are better and to welcome them back into the family. This doesn't mean that they should enable bad behavior of a child and always bail them out of their own mistakes.

Respect should be first learned in the family and it should not be a matter of fear. A parent should not gain respect through punishment of the children, but through example of integrity and family devotion. A child who refuses to do something wrong out of respect for her parents has learned the true nature of respect. I feared misbehaving as a child because I knew I would be punished, but I also feared doing things wrong because I didn't want to disappoint or hurt my parents. The greatest form of respect is to be the best you can be. A true parents shines when their children shine.

Families need to have a foundation of unconditional love. This means that parents and children love each other no matter what the other does. It also means being tough on parents and children through honest criticism. A parent who allows their children to engage in destructive behavior does not love their child. Along with love is compassion, to be compassionate to family members and to show empathy towards others in the family.

Parents need to teach their children about work, hard work which is the keystone of discipline and the ability of children learn to become successful. In the past the entire family had to work together in order to just survive. Today families can get buy doing little or nothing. But the families who are the most successful are the ones who work together and work well together. I can't imagine how children these days can go through life without doing any hard physical labor. Then when they get out on their own it becomes overwhelming to them that they have to do so much work.

It is important that families cook together, garden together, and do projects together. Not only does hard work help with discipline it builds unity within the family, and family members feel that they can trust the other family members. Hard work in families will help with finances, health related issues, and increase the ability for the children to be successful later on in life.

The last principle noted in the Family Proclamation was having wholesome recreational activities. The best part of families is having someone you can go on vacations with, someone you can go on a hike with, and someone you can go to the movies with. There are a lot of great recreational activities families can enjoy doing with each other, and these activities can serve several purposes. They can encourage exercise and learning about the thing that is performed. My fondest memories of my childhood was these family recreational activities especially going on trips to Yellowstone, California, and Washington.

As a family it is important to eat together, pray together, read the scriptures together, work together, and have fun together. It is also important to be able to include family home evening at least once a week for both spiritual instruction and a wholesome family activity. Another common practice is to hold family council meetings to go over what will be happening during the week, upcoming family activities, and discuss major family decisions and finances. It is by doing these activities the family can grow stronger and achieve many goals.

Friends

Many of the same things that involve having a successful family relationship applied to having a successful relationship with friends. The difference between family and friends is that you are not under the same roof as your friends, and the relationship with friends can involve time and distance. You will not see friends as often and they might move which puts strain on the friendship.

It is important to consider all people your friend and attempt to do as Jesus taught and love your neighbor. This involved trust, compassion, forgiveness, repentance, and devotion. A true friend is one who always wants what is best for their friend. This is a good indicator as to how well the friendship is going. If someone is abusive in any form or who does not support and encourage the friend to be there best then the friendship is an unhealthy one.

I have seen too many teens getting into unhealthy relationships with friends who manipulate them and cause them to do things that harm or injure them. This is why peer pressure is so powerful, peer pressure is when someone does something they do not want to do because they are afraid that their peers or friends will not like them anymore and make fun of them. But in the end many teens go down paths they are unable to get out of because of peer pressure. There is a strong need for teens to belong in school, and many will do just about anything to win that acceptance among their peers.

An example of this is when teens join gangs. They have to be jumped into a gang where they are either in the middle of a circle or walk through the members of the gang and are repeatedly kicked, hit, and beaten in order to be part of the gang. Some kids end up in the hospital from getting beaten up. Now I do not know about you, but I think there is a better way to make friends then to get beaten up, and I do not think being hit and kicked by someone makes them a very good friend. In gangs there is a certain level of authority and code that all of the members of the gang have to satisfy. This means that many of the members of the gang are treated like slaves until they earn respect enough from other members of the gang to move up which means hurting other people, and performing criminal activities. All of which is not based on any sense of friendship.

A true friendship would last the test of time and events. Just like in the book of Mormon when Alma the Younger came across the sons of Mosiah and rejoiced because they were still faithful to the gospel. It is when after many years you meet a friend again and it is a joyous one that there is true friendship and that you are willing to help them. Friendship extends into the workplace, school, neighborhood, community, and to strangers. It is a commandment to love on another which includes those that attempt to despitefully use us and to the scary stranger we pass on the street.

Being a friend to all is the toughest thing we have to do on this earth. It is one thing to build relationships and do things with people we enjoy being around and it is another thing to do things for people we cannot stand being around. There are a lot of annoying people with disgusting habits out there. I have come across families who did not ever clean their house and had animals as well in their house it took me everything I could manage to go into the house and clean it without gagging or throwing up. I have come across people who have not taken a shower or bath in months. People who can only put together three word sentences with every other word a swear word.

It is our responsibility to embrace all of these people and to be a friend to them, and by doing so we appreciate our own family and those we care about the most even more. Through our efforts in befriending these people we might be able to spread the gospel and to have them change their lives. The greatest miracle in life is to have someone change their life around. For a person to give up smoking, stop drinking, clean up his language, and to be a more gentle person is a miracle of change.

Coworkers and schoolmates

Another difficult relationship is that of the people you work with or go to school with. Many people are not taught how to get along with others and to work with each other. This is an essential social skill that is critical in life especially when it comes to school and work. Every year, I have students get into groups to complete a group activity and every year students hate being assigned to groups, they want to be in a group with their friends, even as adults when I go to conferences teachers want to be in groups with their friends and not assigned groups.

The key to remember about these situations is that you learn the most when you are with people you do not know. When you are people you know you have already learned about them and how they act in a certain situation. It is a challenge to get to know and befriend those you work with or go to school with you do not like, or only know from afar. These people might have a disgusting habit or have a distasteful personality, but you will be able to learn a lot from these people, and they will help you at your job, and in school if you make the effort to get to know them and become their friends.

Becoming friends doesn't mean that you have to hang out with them all of the time and invite them over to your house, or even do a lot of things for them. It simply means to smile at them every once in a while and make a positive comment on their behalf. It means acknowledging them as human beings and part of your life. You need to find the light of Christ that is within them. Everyone has the light of Christ and some divine quality they poses. It is your responsibility to find what that quality is and to learn from it.

We all have the light of Chris within us and part of God within us, but we also have a little bit of the devil within us as well. It is often easy to see this in others, but difficult to see within ourselves. These are the weaknesses we have that harm ourselves and others. It is important to learn what these weaknesses are and to work on overcoming them. Often it is through others, especially stranger who are able to identify what these weaknesses are. People we do not know well can often give us better honest non-bias feedback about ourselves than someone we are close to.

Charity

"And though I have the gift of prophecy, and understand all mysteries, and all knowledge; and though I have all faith, so that I could remove mountains, and have not charity, I am nothing. And though I bestow all my goods to feed the poor, and though I give my body to be burned, and have not charity, it profiteth me nothing. Charity suffereth long, and is kind; charity envieth not; charity vaunteth not itsel, is not puffed up," (1 Corinthians 13:2-4)

The most important part of social health is Charity or the a pure love of Christ. It is unconditional love in which we do not judge others and love them for who they are. Charity is often associated with acts of kindness and compassion to others. This is a big part of Charity, but Charity can also mean just being a friend to someone who needs a friend, or doing something simple for a neighbor who needs help.

It is important to be able to listen to the spirit and be open on a daily basis for opportunities to help others. Just like the Scout Slogan, "Do a good turn daily," we need to seek out those good turns. They are out there and are part of our daily lives if we are willing to pay attention and recognize when these opportunities come.

Acts of charity could be given to a child, a family member, the elderly, your neighbor, a friend, a co-worker, someone you go to school with, a stranger on the street, it could be even a pet or animal. Remember if you only limit your acts of charity to certain people or just people you lose a lot of opportunities. I have notice that people who are genuine in their kindness to others are also kind and gentle to animals and plants. Kindness is a state of being, and transcends all life. A person who is cruel to animals will be cruel to people.

The way a person treats animals and the people closest to them is a good indicator of how they will treat most people. If you are seeking to be with someone observe how they treat their mother, father, and pets. Then pay attention how they treat you, especially when you make a mistake or when you and that person are in a stressful situation.

Charity is a true form of love and compassion to others. It is something that you need to work on for a lifetime, and even then you might not possess charity in the level of the Savior. It is one quality that if possessed is critical to our eternal progression.

To Do List

1. Be an active listener showing interest and empathy for the speaker
2. Be a better communicator with others sharing your feelings and ideas
3. Have courage in doing what is right saying those things from your heart
4. Be humble and admit to your mistakes and your weaknesses seeking help from others
5. Show charity and compassion towards others with a willingness to serve others even those you may not like.
6. Have integrity and do those things you said you will do.
7. Forgive others and repent of the things you have done that has hurt other people
8. Read the Family a proclamation to the world and follow its teachings
9. Embrace leadership responsibilities and seek to be a good leader to those you are in charge of.
10. Be the person you wish others to be.

Chapter Seven: Financial Health

"But before ye seek for riches, seek ye for the kingdom of God." (Jacob 2:18)

Finances have become a big part of our lives, especially when it comes to financial troubles in our lives. When a person loses his job it not only affects his financial situation, it places a lot of stress on him and his family which in turns causes health problems. There is nothing worse than to be in debt with no means of paying off the debt. There are many things in place to help people who are in debt or have lost their job, but even with these a person's financial situation is important in their lives and in relation to their health.

Tithing and Fast Offerings

"…Those who have thus been tithed shall pay one-tenth of all their interest annually; and this shall be a standing law unto them forever, for my holy priesthood, saith the Lord." (D&C 119:4)

The first thing when it comes to finances would be to seek the kingdom of God which means paying tithing and fast offerings. Not only are these commandments, they come with a set of blessings that come with them if they are obeyed. Many members of the church gain a testimony about tithing and how it has blessed their lives financially.

Paying tithing and fast offerings should be the first thing you do after receiving your paycheck and it should be something that is automatic and done with a spirit gratitude and charity. If you do not have a complete testimony of the law of tithing and do not give freely for fast offerings you need to reexamine your thoughts about money. There are a lot of wealthy people in the world who do not pay tithing or fast offerings, but they are miserable and do not have many of the blessings a person who is living on only a dollar a day and pays his tithing and fast offerings faithfully.

It can be seen as receiving blessings, karma, and the law of abundance which states that there is enough wealth to give to everyone, and if we give freely of our wealth then we will continue to have enough for our means. But if we get into the spirit of pride and selfishness believing that there is only a certain amount of money out there and you need to get as much of it as you can before someone else gets it, you will fall into a trap which leads to unhappiness and despair.

By paying your tithing and fast offerings you get into the proper spirit of money and how it works. It is through tithing that we are able to have nice chapels to meet in each week for church services, and to have activities during the week. It is through tithing that we have nice temples faithful members of the church can attend and do work for the dead. Tithing also supports the church educational system like BYU, the institutes, and seminaries of the world. There are a lot of church functions that would be missing without tithing, and with the tithing that is taken in each month it allows the church to be self sufficient and even one of the wealthiest organizations in the world. No one person or group controls the wealth of the church, but the members of the church share in the wealth collectively.

Fast offerings help to bless the lives of those who are not so fortunate in their lives. It can help a family who has medical expenses they are unable to pay, help a family with the parents are unable to work or have lost their jobs. It helps the homeless and needy and those who have been effected by disasters. The money goes into helping people around the world who are in need. The church works directly with the Red Cross and other organization to help the people around the world, especially when a disaster occurs.

Paying tithing and fast offerings is the first step in financial security and helps to lead into developing a financially sound budget. It also reminds you not to put yourself first when it comes to money and to think of others. There is nothing wrong in being wealthy so long as you are paying your tithing, and a generous fast offering. The wealthy people of the church have helped to make the church strong and to help a lot of people who need help. When it comes to the church and paying tithing and fast offerings everyone is on equal standing. A rich person and a poor person are both seen equally in the eyes of the Lord when it comes to paying their tithing and receiving blessings.

If the only things you do are to pay your tithing, fast offerings, and stay out of debt, you are living a financially secure life and will be blessed tremendously when it comes to money. Even with paying your tithing and fast offerings, you still need to be sensible when it comes to money and not be careless about your spending habits.

Budget

When it comes to financial security, you need to come up with a budget that you review every week and work on. If you do not follow a budget it will be difficult for you to get out of debt, save money, and be financially secure for your future. Budgets are what make businesses and organizations work. Those organizations that follow their budgets rarely get into trouble, but those who do follow their budgets do not go into the red and are able to make a profit or become financially stable.

Budgets consist of two parts the income and the expenses. It is the hope that the income is greater than the expenses. This would result in a profit which could be saved for future use. Because of unexpected expenses and unforeseen events it is important to work towards the goal of saving money on a regular basis. Budgets where the expenses are higher than the income fall apart and cause increased debt and the inability to pay off that debt. So the goal is twofold to increase the income and to reduce the expenses. Always remember when it comes to finances keep the kingdom of God in mind first and then seek after the wealth you desire. First pay your tithing and fast offerings, then pay all necessary bills, and then look at helping your family by getting out of debt which could mean paying off the house or cars you own. Then when you have done all you can for your immediate family, look to helping out your extended family, and other people you might know who need extra financial help.

Income

The obvious income you receive is from your employment. To increase your income you might seek a raise at your job, seek a better paying job or career, look for a second job to work to help out at home financially. In many families both parents work. It is important to make sure that there is at least one parent who is able to be there for children who are still at home and meeting their needs by being their went they come home from school, helping them with school, scouts, young women activities, and other things that children are involved in. It is also important to be able to be there for the family to help teach children the right things in life. This means being there for dinner, family home evening, family counsel, family prayer and scriptures, and being there for wholesome recreational activities.

We live in a society where obtaining things and spending money is encouraged to the point that credit agencies want to lend you money to do things you do not need to do. Instead of paying off our homes people borrow money so that they can buy boats, RVs, and other recreational vehicles. People have more things and have more debt to go with them. This results in both parents working full time with one of the parents having a second job in order to make payments on a credit card that is charging 17% interest.

It is important to increase your income especially if you are attempting to reduce your debt, but you have to look at the overall consequences and implications of working a second job, working long hours, or having your spouse working a lot as well. It might be that you might not be making very much money when you look at childcare, extra money in gas, and other expenses that would relate to having a job. If this is the case then it would be better if you did not work, or work two jobs.

Seek after other ways to get income. If you are able to put money into an IRA, or certificates, or to invest the money then the money will make money through interest. A lot of rich people continue to get richer because they make interest off others. But you have to be consistent in contributing to investments and savings in order to earn enough money to be worth it. It is important to be careful putting a lot of money in the stock market because the money can be earned one day and lost the next. Do not invest money you cannot afford to lose.

Other ways to get money could include doing work at home through the internet, starting up your own part time business that doesn't require a lot of your time like teaching music lessons, or martial art lessons in the neighborhood. The key is to come up with something that people can use or need and are willing to pay money for, and that you have a ready market with several families who would be interest. Just like with the stock market, it is important to do your research and to look at the costs it would take to start your own business from home.

You might also contract out your services to schools or businesses in something you specialize in, or that you make furniture or art that you can sell to a local store who will sell them to their customers. The key is to be able to make money in such a way that does not take you away from your family and makes you excited and happy about what you are doing and is helping you out with extra income. If the time and money you spend on a financial venture is greater than what you are making, it might not be such a smart idea.

It is important to look to the future to see if your income will meet needs in the future. You know that bills will continue to go up, but you might also have children to put through college or send on a mission. This would mean that you will need to increase your income, and if you know that your job will not be paying you what you need, you will have to plan on getting a different job, or a second job in order to pay for the future expenses.

My mother went to work full time before I went on a mission in order to help pay for my mission and to put money in my savings account for college when I got back home. This helped me on my mission as well helped to pay for my college since I did not have any scholarships and I did not qualify for a grant.

You may need to look at education and further training in order to be able to make more money in the future. If you become complacent when it comes to your job, you might end up losing your job because you haven't kept up to date on the latest breakthroughs or technology for your work. Education and skills training is often an ongoing process in order to continue to move up in your job. So it is important to plan for the future and seize the opportunities for further training and educational opportunities.

Expenses

Expenses come into two categories those things that are essential and those things that are not essential or in other words the things you need and the things you want. The first thing to do would be to look at all of the bills you have and those things you cannot live without. This is one way to save a lot of money and to take a look at your real budget. If your bills are more than your income then there is a serious problem, and you will have to take a detailed look at your bills and start to trim down those things you can live without.

You cannot go without paying the house payment, car payment, gas and electricity, or phone. You will also have insurance automobile, home, and medical that you will not be able to live without. But there are some bills you might be able to trim or get rid of. For example you might get rid of your land line and just use your cell phones, or you might get rid of your cell phones. I remember when it was shocking to get a $30.00 phone bill and yet we spend over $100.00 a month on cell phone charges. Saving $100.00 a month is a lot, and people lived without cell phones for centuries. You might even find you have time to do a lot more things in your life and have a lot less stress if you gave up your cell phone. This may not be practical for people who use their cell phone for work, but for most of us, cell phones are more of a convenience then a necessity. Believe me I have live without my cell phone, and I believe I would be better without it.

You might look into having only one car as well. You can save a lot in gas, insurance, and maintenance by only having one car. If you can ride a bike or walk to work you not only save a lot of money, you get exercise as well. Most of the people in the world do not own a vehicle. In some cases you might be able to save money riding public transportation, but this can also be a great expense unless you get rid of a vehicle so that you do not have to pay for the insurance.

Bills can be cut in half by practicing energy saving practices which means using less water, gas, and electricity. This will require some sacrifice and research into what will work and what you and your family will be able to do. You can also look into investing into alternative power sources like solar and wind. These can be expensive, but in the long run they might prove to save you a lot of money especially in areas where gas and electricity are expensive.

Other bills that you might consider cutting might be magazine subscriptions, newspaper subscriptions, organizational dues, clubs, or other things you might belong to and do not need. You just have to examine the bills you have and decide if you can live without them or not. Those you can live without might be worthy of getting rid of. It might be hard to part form a magazine or organization you have belong to for years, but when it comes to your finances it is the best thing to do.

Once you have gone through your essential bills you have each month, you will then need to look at the other essentials such as groceries, medical expenses, and things that come up like getting tires for the car, or replacing the refrigerator. These things you need to spend money on, but they can sometimes cause you to go into the red for the month, and they can sometimes be on the border line between need and want.

Take a look at how much money you spend on groceries each month and you might be surprised at how much you can cut from that by looking at what you need and what you want. You can also do some research as to which stores are cheaper than others and the quality of products you buy. When you buy food it is important to buy healthy foods and those foods that will help you and your family be healthy first, and then it is important to budget some money for food storage, and then you can buy some treat or dessert, but only sparingly. You might be surprised at how much money you can save if you just cut out all of the food you do not need, and cut down on the quantity of food you buy.

Remember that the processed packaged foods are the most unhealthy for you and can be the most expensive to buy as well. Make sure to buy sufficient quantities of food that is healthy for you and food that can go a long way such as rice, and whole grains. Generic brands are just as good as the brand named products, but do not just shop by price. I remember buying a lot of food items that were on sale, but regretting it because the food was something that we normally did not eat and it was also not healthy for us. I have fallen for the trap of buying a lot of ice cream because it was on sale. It is okay to buy treats now and then, but to buy too much is a waste of money and will make you unhealthy.

You will find that you can save a lot of money over $100.00 by going through your grocery budget and only purchasing those things you need. When it comes to wants you it is important to prioritize them as well, and ask yourself why you want this item. If it is something that will benefit you and your family then it could be something worth saving for. You should not go into debt for anything except for a house and a car, and even with these you need to buy within your needs and not purchase a home or car you cannot afford and will put a lot of stress on your financial situation.

There might be a vacation you want to go on. It is important to put money aside for the vacation and do some research as to how much money you can save while you are on the vacation with reserving a hotel, car rental, and airfare to your destination. Make sure that you save up enough money for the vacation and have a budget you stick buy so that you do not go into debt for the vacation.

You need to save money for presents and celebrations you might have. Attempt to reduce the amount of money you spend on presents, and you might even work out a deal with your relatives that you choose families, or just exchange cards for birthdays in order for everyone to save money. It can be a great financial burden for people who feel obligated to buy presents for their family, their relatives, and all other persons they know. Christmas is the biggest time of the year for businesses to earn money from costumers, but it is also the time of year when people tend to spend more money than they normally do going into debt. The Christmas spirit as well as the joy is gone and people feel miserable at how much money they spent on toys that will break and be forgotten, and trivial gifts that people will not life and disregard.

I think it is ironic that we give a gift to get a gift and we feel a sense of responsibility to give a gift that the person would be wowed by. It become a competition as to who will give the best gift to someone. Children get caught up with the media spirit of the holidays and expect to be given expensive gifts for the holidays and are disappointed with what they get. Whatever happened to giving gifts that are made and come from the heart?

Becoming financially self sufficient and secure is not all that complicated and once you have looked at your income and expenses and came up with a budget you will be able to be more at ease with your financial situation. It is important to be able to review your budget on a weekly basis looking at income and expenses. This will give you an opportunity to see the things you bought and to look at those things you bought you needed and those things you bought because you wanted them. You will be able to make adjustments in your budget and be able to learn from your mistakes.

I learned the hard way that it is important to do some research into a company before seeking their services. We had raccoons living in our chimney a mother and her babies. I knew we had to get rid of them, so I called animal control who referred me to another company. The entire process resulted in me paying over $800.00 to get rid of the raccoons. If I had known this beforehand I would have never went with the company. It was one of those financial moments I had learned a great deal into researching other companies that perform the same service. The only problem was that the selection of companies that did this service was slim, but I could have done other things to get rid of the raccoons instead of having to go through all of that with the company.

Financial health takes a lot of planning and research. It is a dynamic area of your health that is constantly changing and will need attention just like the rest of your health. If you neglect it, you will lose the integrity of your finances and there would be financial collapse. Make sure to pay your tithing, fast offerings and bills first and then looks at your needs and wants for the rest of your budget attempting to save some money each month and to pay down your debt.

There are many other ways you can save money. Entertainment is often a big money pit in which you can spend a lot of money going to movies and getting entertainment in your lives. One very easy way to save money would be to make your local library your best friend. You can barrow movies and books at the library and even use the internet for free. This means you can do away with your television service, internet service, and become smarter and more refined by using the time and money you would have spent on entertainment on the library services. You can get your entertainment through reading and watching movies you get from the library. You can even find programs and many other things that are offered at the local library that can satisfy your entertainment cravings.

Many communities will also have free entertainment possibilities especially if you have children. This is one reason why parents take their children to parades, because they are free, and they throw out free candy to the children. You can watch fireworks, attend Easter egg hunts, and local concerts all free of charge. Some communities have free zoos and other places in which families can go to. You can go on nature hikes, go to the local park, and many other things for entertainment without having to pay for expensive tickets. This will help you to make better decisions about your money and what you spend it on.

Many people who have a lot of money are protective of their money and do not spend it on frivolous items. It just does not make any sense to go into debt over things you do not need and to pay the extra interest on your credit card. Save money and invest it wisely and you will be able to have be at peace with your finances and not stressed out about paying your bills or coming up with the money to pay for the house payment and worried that you will lose your car, house, or family when it comes to finances as being the number one reason why couples separate.

To Do List

1. Pay your tithing and fast offerings every month without delay
2. Work on developing a budget
3. Look at ways to increase your income
4. Look at ways to decrease your expenses
5. Examine the wants and needs of your expenses and concentrate on only spending money for those things you need.
6. Get as much education and skills training as you can
7. Keep up to date on your job and ways you can be promoted
8. Replace your entertainment budget with the library and public events that are free
9. Review your budget on a weekly basis.
10. Reduce your holiday and gift spending.

Chapter Eight: Environmental Health

"When we heal the earth, we heal ourselves,"
David Orr

One aspect of health that is often overlooked is our environmental health. Even with the emphasis on global warming and taking care of the environment many people do not consider taking care of the environment in terms of their own health. It is something that is talked of on television and in the news from time to time when there is an oil spill in the ocean or there is an endangered species that is about to go extinct, or scientists try to explain the change in weather patterns.

We do not have to have a Ph.D. or be an expert on the environment to know what is happening to our environment and how it affects our health. All you have to do is to jog along a busy street and breath in the exhaust of the cars and trucks that go buy to know that what you are breathing in is not a good thing. In Utah alone the population has tripled over the past twenty years and with it the air quality and pollution has gone way up. Just looking out on a clear day you can see the brown haze that blankets the sky.

Even in areas like St. George, Utah there is evidence of air pollution. Some areas as remote as the four corners area there is poor air quality. It is disturbing to go to a National Park and to look at a sign from a lookout that shows a distant mountain range that you cannot see anymore and reading the sign it reveals that the visibility is no longer possible because of the air pollution, and this is far away from any large city.

Along the Wasatch Front in Utah there are several valleys that create a bowl and trap polluted air and it is only when a strong storm comes in that the air is forced from the valley for a short period of time. Then it returns and hangs out for several weeks before another storm comes in. Since it Utah does not get a lot of storms and is a dry state there is a lot of air pollution that remains for long periods of time. Not only is it not pretty to look at, the air pollution is affecting people's health especially the young and old. More children are getting asthma and allergies than before due to the air quality.

If Utah which is one of the least populated states is feeling the effects of how we are treating the environment then you can imagine how bad places like California, Texas, and New York are with millions of more people living in those states. Every time I have visited New York City the largest in the United States, I have gotten a headache within minutes of entering the city and have that headache for several days until I get used to the pollution.

The water quality in many places in Utah and the United States is not as healthy as it should be. Most of the water is drinkable, but may contain enough contaminants to be concerned about long term exposure to the water that is coming into people's homes. The increase in population also increases the consumption of water and with the higher usage of water the less water we will have which poses more problems in the future with water shortages.

If we are to look at America as terms of the environment and the coming of the industrial revolution we can see that we have improved in some areas, but have gotten worse in others. Our factories are cleaner than in the past, we use natural gas instead of wood or coal to heat our homes which is a lot cleaner. Just stand outside a building that uses coal to heat it and you can tell an immediate difference.

There is nothing worse than to see the black smoke from the burning of coal and to smell the burnt coal. My first teaching job was at an old school that still used coal to heat the building. My classroom was unfortunately right next to the boiler. Each morning I would enter a blackened

157

room filled with coal smoke. I feared of getting black lung disease from the two years I worked there. The football field would also be filled with smoke when they started to burn the coal in the fall when the weather changed. It was a chocking smell that caused me to gag. I was pleased that I got a job somewhere else and did not have to breathe in the coal smoke anymore. If everyone used coal to heat their homes the valleys would be black with smoke and people would end up dying each year as they did in London when people used coal there to heat their homes.

With an emphasis on taking care of the environment we have done a better job of protecting the land and making sure not to put trash everywhere and to not poison the water by dumping toxins into the water supply. The areas we have failed at is to come up with zero emission cars that are affordable and practical to the consumers. We also are not doing as well as many countries when it comes to the waste we produce each year. Americans produce more waste than any other country in the world. We are consumers and as we consume we produce a lot of garbage. It is growing increasingly more difficult to come up with areas to put our trash, and with the increase of population there will be an increase in waste produced.

It seems like there are more recycling programs and cities are starting to have recycling programs that greatly reduce the trash produced by people. But the real problem is that it seems like we are years behind where we should be in terms of dealing with population growth and the pollution that is involved with it. We cannot keep up with all of the cars that are on the road and the amount of carbon that is put into the air. It will take not just big business and government to solve the problem. It will take all of the consumers to demand environmentally friendly cars and products that will help to not only be safer for the environment, but that which will help clean up the environment as well.

Just think about how much cleaner the air would be if instead of polluting the air, cars actually cleaned up air. It would be like riding a tree to work. The idea sounds a little crazy, but it is what we will need to do in the future unless we want to spend more money on health care and do not worry about cancer, heart disease, and asthma. Something needs to be done with the millions of cars out there that are polluting the environment. Unfortunately I believe that it will be too late and it may get to the point where we will not be able to reverse the damage we have already caused. I would like to be able to have a world in which my great grandchildren will be able to enjoy and not be getting sick all of the time.

Homes

The first place we can make into a safe environment is our homes. We spend each night and many days inside our homes which makes it critical that the environment is not only safe but healthy for us. A healthy home can make up for an unhealthy area. You can do many things to make your home healthy and to ensure that you and your children are healthy.

First you should make the air quality in your home safe to breathe. You may need to get your air tested to see if there are any toxic fumes in the air you and your family are breathing. Then you need to get a good furnace, and make sure that your ducts are clean. My wife and I moved into an older home where the couple who lived there smoked. Needless to say we replaced all of the duct work and the furnace that was top of the line meaning that it was not only more fuel efficient it was healthier.

It is important to get a good quality filter that filters all of the contaminants in the air. There are also UV lights that you can place in your furnace that will kill just about all of the bacteria and viruses that may get into the air. The air quality in your home can mean the difference between getting sick several times a year, to not getting sick at all. It may be more expensive, but it is well worth it. You can save a lot of money in the long run in doctor's visits, and time lost at work and at school.

A healthier home environment makes it so that you feel better eating dinner together as a family, having family home evening, and doing things at home together thinking about how healthy your home is. Newer homes may have less toxins, but many of the homes have less than adequate heating and air conditioning when it comes to air quality. Older homes may need more extensive renovation when it comes to replacing ducts that cannot be cleaned and a furnace that may be a death trap waiting to happen.

Water is also another area of concern. You can also have your water tested in your home. Some older homes may have lead or other toxins in the water because of old pipes, and the ground water in some areas might be contaminated. Most water that comes into the homes are safe enough to drink, but you may want to take an added precaution by filtering the water you are drinking. Most basic filters will filter out all of the bacteria and germs that will get you sick, but you have to get a more advanced filter to get rid of viruses that are in the water.

Just making sure you have clean air to breathe and clean water to drink makes a huge difference in your health. There are many other things you can do to improve your environment at your house, by making sure it is cleaned on a regular basis and that you are using environment friendly cleaning products. Washing your clothes and making sure things are tidy and clean to kill germs that are brought into the house.

Another aspect of health and the environment is known as Feng Shui meaning wind and water is the science and art of placement of objects in the home to harness nature's energy and to make the environment a healthy place to live in. You do not have to be an expert on Feng Shui to appreciate how you feel in a place that is pleasing to look at. Make your home and your yard a place of beauty that you enjoy looking at and living in.

If you think your home and yard are ugly and you hate living there it will definitely affect your health, but if you enjoy your home and yard and love how it looks you will have better overall health. It all goes to the positive and negative energy you have at your home. Just like how the temples are a place of peace we can make our homes the same way. You might not be able to capture the complete atmosphere you feel at the temple in your home, but you can come close.

"Set in order your houses; keep slothfulness and uncleanness far from you." (D&C 90:18)

By keeping your house in order and making sure that everyone in the house has a task to do to make sure the house stays in order will help to free up valuable time to do other things with the family such as fun activities doing art, playing games, playing musical instruments, going on a hike and so forth.

In the yard to help your home you can make sure you have trees, and plants that help to clean the environment. You can grow a flower garden as well as a vegetable garden with several plants that will come up each year that will enhance the beauty of your yard. There is nothing better to be able to go outside and enjoy your backyard. It can be relaxing and release a lot of the stress and anxiety you may have built up over the day.

Work and School

We also spend a lot of time at work and school. These areas can also have a great influence on our health as well. Strive to make sure air and water quality are good, and the area is tidy and clean. Another important factor at work and school is to make the environment as stress free as possible. In some cases this is difficult to do, but you can start with what you can do and then give suggestions to others to help with the environment. It may take repainting and repairing the environment to make it look better. It may take the removal of toxins from the environment in order to make it safe. There are still many old buildings that have lead paint, asbestos ceiling and floor tiles.

By changing the environment it will change the way people interact with each other and you might find a change in attitude and people will be more positive than how they were before. People work better when they are in an atmosphere they feel better in than an atmosphere that is ugly and falling apart. I always wondered why in some schools they have ugly orange carpet or other ugly areas of the school. Those things not only cause distress among the students, but it makes for an unhealthy learning environment for the children who are disturbed by the color and thus stressed to the point that they have a hard time concentrating on the learning that is supposed to be taking place.

Work and school should be a place that feels comfortable and relaxing to be in. If the atmosphere is stressful and unhealthy then it will greatly affect your health, and you should consider improving the atmosphere or finding a different place to work at or go to school at. This was the greatest argument for desegregation in schools, because the schools white children were going to were better than those African American children were going to. The atmosphere was so much better and it was affecting the learning environment and how much the children learned.

Even today there are many schools who are in desperate need of a change in environment. Schools are not equal by any means. The schools in wealthy neighborhoods are in better condition and receive more donations to keep up the school and the atmosphere at the school than those schools that are in poor neighborhoods. This is another reason why there are some schools kids hate to go to and carry with them a negative attitude towards the school thus effecting their learning than other schools where students are excited about attending.

The same goes with businesses as well. Some businesses people love to work for and others it becomes a temporary stop before moving on to another job. Successful businesses and schools take the time and money to invest in the environment. It is important not to sit idly by and wait for your environment to change, you need to put forth the effort to make a difference and help to change it yourself.

Neighborhood and Community

Your neighborhood and community are just as important as your home and where you work. It is where you live and it can affect your health in many different ways. Chances are the water you drink and the air you breathe when you go outside is part of your community. If you life in a big city there are a lot of things that will influence your health and environment. Not only do you have to be concerned out the environment you need to be concerned with crime and poverty in your community as well.

The ideal would be that everyone in the community works together to make sure that everyone in the community is health, safe, and they work on making sure that they protect the environment. Neighborhoods can have neighborhood watches, can have recycling programs, and beautify their community through planting trees and flowers. If the community works together then they can grow closer together and be able to solve any problems they might have.

Health tends to be a result of the environment we live in and if it is an unhealthy environment we become unhealthy along with it. It isn't any wonder that when it comes to life expectancy that the lowest is in Harlem New York, and the highest in the United States is in places like Montana, Utah, and Oregon places where there is not a lot of people and the atmosphere is a lot better than that of New York, Chicago, and Los Angeles.

Reduce, Reuse, and Recycle

We can follow the principles of reduce, reuse, and recycle in our homes, work, and community. The idea is to reduce the amount of trash we produce, this can also help to reduce the amount of food we eat making it so that we lose weight or do not gain unnecessary pounds. You can keep track of how much food you eat and reduce a little bit of it each day. You can also reduce the amount of water you use by taking shorter showers, and eliminating the amount of other things you use on a regular basis which will be better for the environment, help you to save money, and make your life less stressful.

Reusing things has been a habit for people who grew up during the depression. Everyone knows a parent or grandparent who saves containers to use for something else. This is important because there are a lot of containers we throw away each week that we could use for something else. It reduces the amount of trash that is in the bump and it allows for you to save money and use the item for something else.

You can be very creative in reusing things for something else you do. I found that many of the plastic food containers that I got were perfect to use for paint containers for my art. Craft stores charge a lot of money for paint containers, and are not very good, while I found that if I just cleaned out the food containers, I could use them to keep the paint I was using for a painting. I saved a lot of money and I did not add more junk to the garbage dump that would take more than a hundred years to decompose. These containers I could use indefinitely with the projects I have.

There are a lot of containers that could be used as planters for flowers or vegetables. Many containers can also be used as storage containers for odds and ends that you might collect or store for future use. So the next time you think about throwing away something think about if you can reuse it to do something else with.

Recycling has been around for a very long time. I remember collecting aluminum cans to sell to the recycling place. Since then cities have developed their own recycling programs. There are many stores that will recycle bottles and shopping bags. You can make sure to do research in your own area and start to recycle some of the items at your home such as plastic, paper, glass, and metal. You can get to the point that you can reduce your trash by half or more. You might even be able to make some money by recycling some of the items.

Another thing you can get into the habit of doing is to mulch. You can use some of your table scraps like fruits, vegetables, and grains that you can put in your mulching bin. This can then be used to help fertilize your flowers and vegetables the healthy way. Through reducing, reusing, recycling, and mulching you can just about eliminate your waste and live a healthier live by making your environment healthier.

Leave No Trace

Another thing to consider when protecting the environment is to protect it when you venture into the outdoors and go camping. All outdoor areas have their own set of regulations and attempt to enforce them such as

National Parks where you have to abide by the regulations or get a hefty fine. In Yellowstone you cannot leave food on a picnic table because it will attract animals like bears to the area. You cannot take anything from a National Park like a stone or a flower. Certain areas may be off limits to cars, and other motor vehicles in order to protect just environments.

Even with all of the regulations there are many areas that are impacted by the millions of people who visit our National Parks, National Forests, BLM lands and state parks each year. With the amount of people who go to these places it is important that each do their part in protecting and preserving the land. Without this it will destroy the land and make it so that the beautiful areas I saw as a child will be there for my grandchildren.

Leave No Trace is a set of principles to follow while in the wilderness areas to help protect the environment. They were founded by those who have seen the impact of humans in the wilderness areas and have developed these set of principles or ethics to help preserve the land. There are seven principles that if followed will help to preserve the environment in such a way that there will be little impact or no trace left of your presence. They are to plan and prepare before entering going into the wilderness by learning about regulations and not going at peak times of the year as well as planning on what food to bring and how to cook it. Camping and traveling on durable surfaces is important to not damage the plant life. This means staying on trails and not making trails or altering the environment to make a good campsite. Disposing of waste properly or bring out all trash and if there is not a restroom nearby digging a cat hole and burring human waste, being careful with fire using existing fire pits, and not making another one, and making a fire that will not leave a trace by placing dirt underneath and using small pieces of wood that will burn to ashes and not be left as a scare on the land.

You should leave what you find and not take out things to hang up in your home. This means that fossils and pretty rocks are left for others to enjoy where they are found. It also means that you preserve the history of the area by not talking out historical evidence. I remember going on a trail in Moab where I saw a set of dinosaur tracks in the slickrock. It was one of the most exciting things I have ever seen because it was exactly where the dinosaur had made them and not in a museum where they could have been altered or copied. It is so much better to experience things where they happened and not in a museum.

We need to all respect others when we are camping and the wildlife in the area so that we do not cause them to get used to humans or change their lifestyle that will injure their existence or interfere with those who go in the wilderness after us. There are more people who are injured or attacked by animals in the wilderness because the animals are getting used to human contact, and people are getting careless when they see animals. When entering parks such as Yellowstone National Park there are signs that take about how you should treat the animals.

In Yellowstone you are not to feed any animals and for bears and bison you should not be less than 100 yards from them. They also have restrictions on where to store food and not to leave food out which would attract animals. I remember a boy who was dragged out of his tent by a bear and killed because he had food smell on his clothes from eating dinner that night. There was a story of scouts who left food in their tent and mice got into their tent and their food. You are coming into the home of the animals, it is important to respect and to abide by the regulations of the places you visit.

Preparing for the Outdoors

It is important to be prepared when going into the outdoors which is part of being healthy. This means protecting yourself from the sun by covering up and applying sunscreen to areas of your skin that will be exposed to the sun. Overexposure to the sun for repeated periods of time can result in skin cancer. It is also not fun to get a sun burn. I do not like putting a lot of chemicals on my skin so I just cover up with a long sleeved shirt, pants, a hat, and polarized sun glasses so that I can see better while out in the sun.

Many people might think I am crazy trekking around in the desert wearing pants and a long sleeved shirt. But in actuality I am just as cool as the other people, because the shirts I wear are thin and allow the breeze to go through to my skin thus cooling me. I do not have to worry about all of the sunscreen, insect repellent, and getting scrapes or cuts on my arms or legs. The best part is that I can go for a long time and not get too hot or exhausted. In the fall and spring my hiking wardrobe doesn't change, and in the winter time I add some extra layers. I rarely wear cotton except at home, because it soaks up sweat and traps it against the skin making me sticky in the summer and cold in the winter.

It is also important that whenever hitting the trail no matter what season it is to bring some water and some salty snacks. This will help you to retain water and not get dehydrated. If you just drink water it could make you sick, by flushing out all of the salt and sodium from your body that you need. Sport drinks can be okay if you do not drink too much of them, because they give you the salt, water, and potassium along with some sugar that your body could use.

Get to know your limits and your skill level whenever you are traveling to places, and make sure to get to know the place you are at especially if you have never been there before by getting maps of the area along with detailed descriptions of hikes and things you should know and bring to the hike.

Exploring the outdoor on hikes is just about the healthiest thing you can enjoy doing. It will increase your heart rate and give the exercise you need. It provided beautiful scenery, cleaner air, and nature sounds all of which will calm and relieve stress. Hiking helps to stimulate the mind at all of the different things you can see. Plus hiking will get you nearer to God. Why do you think that God spoke with Moses, Nephi, and many others in the mountains. There are many sacred places on the earth, other than the temple mountains and wilderness areas are the among those sacred places.

Many cultures have built things on the mountains as part of this sacred ritual. There are monasteries in the mountains of Tibet, and Nepal. In Wyoming there is an ancient medicine wheel on the top of a mountain. Many cultures look at the mountains near their homes as the home to the Gods. Even the Greeks believed that the Gods lived on Mt. Olympus. John Muir when he started to feel melancholy or sick took off for the mountains of California to get better. I have done the same.

There is just something about the mountains and the hikes I have been on that renews my body, mind, and spirit. I just have to respect nature and make sure that it is still there for my grandchildren and their children. If we allow our environment to be polluted and chocked with toxins not only will the plants and animals die, but we will soon follow. It says in the last days that the Earth will be cleansed by fire or have a baptism of fire. Forest fires have helped to clean and rejuvenate the forests, only we have spent a decade of repressing the fires that many of the forest are infected and thousands of trees and other plant life are dying.

It is sad to see all of the trees that have died because of a beetle that would have been killed by forest fires. I am not sure when it will take place, but because of all of the destruction of the environment it will have to heal itself through fire. With decades of mismanagement with the forest service and the advancement of people into the wilderness areas it is increasingly difficult for us to keep our wilderness areas healthy.

It is our responsibility to help to preserve and protect our forests and our wilderness areas just like it is our responsibility to protect our families and our communities. The wilderness area are just as much part of our health as the air we breathe, because a lot of the clean air and water come from the wilderness areas of the world. The life giving water that flows into Pakistan, India, Nepal, Tibet, and Bangladesh comes from the Himalayas. The water that sustains all of the west and Great Plains comes from the Rocky Mountains, and in the East it is the Appalachian Mountains. The mighty Amazon comes from the Andes, and many other areas of the world get their water from the mountains and the wilderness areas. It is the trees of the world that clean and replenish the air of the world, this is why scientists are concerned with the cutting down of the forests of the Amazon and tropical regions of the world.

History has proven that the destruction of an ecosystem often has disastrous effects on the environment. There are countless plants, animals, and cultures that have been forced into extinction. In recent times we have been more conscious about this, and have taken measures to ensure protection of many of the endangered species on the earth, but there is still a lot of threat to many animals and plants some of which are unknown to man.

To Do List

1. Make sure that the air you are breathing in your home is healthy with an adequate filter, furnace, duct work, and possibly even have a UV filter installed with your furnace.
2. Filter the water you drink in your home and have it tested for toxins
3. Make your home and your yard stress free and a place where you can relax and enjoy just being there. Make it beautiful and practice some Feng Shui
4. Take pride in your neighborhood and community and make it a safe beautiful place to live.
5. Practice Reduce, Reuse, Recycle, and Mulch to cut down on the waste you produce.
6. Make it a point to practice Leave No Trace principles in the wilderness and take the time to respect and protect the environment.
7. Be part of the environment by taking walks around your community on a regular basis and take part in community activities.
8. Each year venture into the wilderness areas to enjoy God's creations and the beauty of the world. Many of the most beautiful places on earth are in Utah, and the geothermal wonder of the world is in Yellowstone. There are many other wonderful places throughout the world.
9. Find your special place, a place that is in nature that makes you feel closer to God and nature. It might be in your back yard, or at a local park, or it might be on a favorite hike you go on.

10. Make it a point to be prepared when going outside to cover up and use sunscreen. Drink water and eat salty snacks. Dress for the weather and be aware of the possible dangers of the area. Respect wildlife and obey the regulations of the area.

Chapter Nine: Living a Healthy Life

"To keep the body in health is a duty, otherwise we shall not be able to keep our mind strong and clear," Buddha

I hope that his book has taught you that there are a lot of things that are involved in your overall health and that these things are interconnected. If one area of your health suffers the rest of your health will be affected by it. This is why as Latter Day Saints it is critical that we pay attention to our health. We often see health as something that is just part of the Word of Wisdom or something that only fanatical people work on, or a passing fancy where we will get to it when we have the time or when we are not so busy and we can dedicate a couple of months to losing the pounds we want to lose.

Health can be a lifelong struggle, it is one of those lessons in life we must learn and must control. It is no wonder that the biggest challenge in our life is our bodies and that we came to the earth to receive a body so that we can learn to deal with it and all of the things that goes with it. If you just look at the body you can see that not only health is the central part of its existence it involves all of the aspects of health including the spiritual realm. Just think of many of the temptations and sins that have brought down people which involve the body. There are the obvious ones of sexuality, substance abuse, and overindulgence of food. Many of the other sins are just extensions of these.

Murder is often a result of some love triangle involving sexual relations, substance abuse often leads to lying stealing, and injury of other people. Over eating can lead to more stress in a person's life which can propel a person to do things they would not normally do such as spend too much money on food and other items, neglect responsibilities and become idle with no motivation to work or support his family.

Many of the temptations that come into the mind involve physical desires and cravings. Even greed and the desire to have more money is physical in the sense that when we think of becoming rich our minds release endorphins and adrenaline to make us feel pleasure in wanting to become rich causing people to do things that they would never think about doing, but because of this desire to be rich is so strong they ignore their own sense of morality.

The worst part of these desires are that they can never be satisfied and if left unchecked will overcome the person and force them to commit more sins and crimes. It is only through having overall health that we are better able to withstand these temptations and have better control over our life. Just like in the beginning of section 89 of the Doctrine and Covenants where the Lord says that the Word of Wisdom is a warning to us to be able to withstand the evil designs of men. It sends a message for our overall health. If we are healthy we are better able to withstand the temptations of Satan and become closer to the Lord.

By taking just one aspect of health we might be able to see how health can help us become more spiritual. Exercise can help to get the body in shape. Through Exercise you can develop discipline and because of the increase in blood supply you get more oxygen to the brain and you will be able to think more clearly. By having more discipline and being able to think more clearly you will be able to see temptations for what they are and will be able to push them to the side and replace them with virtuous thoughts. Exercise will also allow you to be able to listen to your body and spirit better as well as the promptings of the Holy Ghost.

If you are having problems with your spirituality and find it difficult to read the scriptures and say your prayers, you might want to go out for walks, and start an exercise routine, because it will help you to be able to read the scriptures and say your prayers without having the difficulty of trying to understand the scriptures and have well organized thoughts when you say your prayers.

Those you do not exercise will start to have health problems, and even minor health concerns will effort their spirituality. Lack of exercise can result in headaches, muscle strains, and poor mental judgment which could lead a person to be more susceptible to temptations and make it difficult to pray, read scriptures, and attend church meetings as well as full filing callings.

Being healthy is something we must strive to achieve and make part of our lifestyle. It is through this healthy lifestyle we are able to be stronger physically, mentally, and spiritually. Just like how we have made brushing our teeth a habit, we should make reading scriptures, praying, and jogging as part of your life. Plan on eating healthy meals, exercising, financial planning, making your home beautiful, and working on family council and activities that are engaging and learning to those involved.

It has been hard for me to write a book about health, because I do not want it to be like all of the other health books where there is a set exercise routine, diet, and program you would follow. It would be against everything I believe for me to just give you a set program to follow when you are different than I am and what I do is tailored for me, and something I have taken a lifetime to prefect. What I do with exercise, diet, spiritual growth, sleep, and social interactions is something I have made for my own lifestyle something I can do for the rest of my life.

You need to come up with your own healthy diet, exercise routine, sleep habits, social interaction, and spiritual routine. There are so many things involved when it comes to these areas of health that you have to figure those things out. It will take you a long time to figure those things out and part of the journey in figuring all of these things out will be the growth and learning that you will need to be able to get back to your Heavenly Father. I have attempted to steer you in the right direction and lay a foundation for you to be able to start changing your lifestyle. But it does have to come from you and you need to make it your own. You cannot follow someone else's routine or program. I have tried it all my life, but it just doesn't work. Sure you will see some results and it will motivate you to continue with the program a little longer, but a few weeks, months, or years you will abandon the program because it is not part of who you are.

It is like how I got into doing taekwondo. I liked the school I went to and my master. I feel that it was right for me, and also got into tai chi, yoga, and Aikido. But you might find that you prefer karate, judo, or other martial arts. You might not even like doing martial arts and just simply do some yoga. It is what you find you enjoy the most, what will fit into your lifestyle and what the spirit guided you to do.

I am convinced that the Holy Ghost has guided me to get my black belt in taekwondo. I also believe it was inspiration when I got involved with yoga and tai chi when I did. Each thing I have put into my lifestyle has improved it. There are times I am happier and feel better than I did when I was much younger. I am convinced that I am healthier than I was before, because I have found these things to be miracles in my life.

If it wasn't for exercise and health in my life, I would have been dead long ago from heart disease. Without exercise I would have become obese quickly and would have gotten high blood pressure which would eventually have lead to heart disease and an early untimely death. But because of my healthy lifestyle I was able to get married in the temple and have a child. I have been able to experience happiness, I never thought was possible. I have been able to teach and influence countless numbers of students in the schools I have been at.

Do not let poor health interfere with your spirituality and your quality of life. Do not allow yourself to continue to have poor health habits and allow it to affect your callings at church and your responsibilities at home with your family. A great deal of happiness rests on your health, make the most of it. Think about living a life free of pain, free from suffering, and with the ability to do just about anything you want physically, mentally, and spiritually. Think of the windows of heaven being opened up to you and you receiving more blessings that you are able to accept in this life.

A successful life and a healthy life starts with you. You need to take the first step in making a difference in your life. It will be hard to do, but once you get started and see the results it will be the motivation you need to be able to complete a healthy lifestyle that will work for you and will be something you will be able to do the rest of your life.

The thing you have to keep in mind the entire time is how even though physical, spiritual, and mental health are separate they are also the same in terms of health. Just like the Godhead and how Heavenly Father, Jesus Christ, and the Holy Ghost are separate individuals they make up the Godhead and act as one God and have one purpose in bringing to pass our exaltation and eternal life. All aspects of health in your life have one purpose and that is to make you healthier and be able to do those things that will bring about the most joy and happiness in your life.

In order to see Jesus and Heavenly Father you need to be filled with the Holy Ghost, and in order to get to the Father you have to go through Jesus Christ. All of them act as one and yet they all have their own mission they have to fulfill. The aspects of our health are the same they all act to help the other, but have their own separate mission as well.

It is your responsibility to learn out how they are interrelated and what each of their missions are.

When I exercise and I am thinking about my exercise, I am able to not only have the blood flow faster through my veins and strengthen my heart and lungs, I am able to connect with my body and get in tune with my spirit. When I am in tune with my spirit, I am closer to the Holy Ghost and am able to listen to the promptings of the Holy Ghost better. It is harder for me to listen to the Holy Ghost when I am laying on the couch watching television or when I am binging on some snacks.

By connecting with the spiritual side of things along with the physical and using mental concentration exercise, eating, and all other aspects of health goes to a higher plain or level of existence that is hard to describe, but once it is experienced it becomes a part of you. When I go out jogging, I am not just going out jogging. I feel my heart beating, the air as it fills my lungs, and the energy as it flows through my body. I feel my spirit as it connects with my body and have a prayer in my heart as I communicate with my Father in Heaven and for a brief moment I am able to touch all aspects of my health. My mind becomes clear, my thoughts are virtuous with not just means clean and pure, but also means power. For a time I experience a power or energy that goes far beyond just an adrenaline rush.

There are times when I have ran that it feels as if I am floating above the ground and am not just moving my legs as they pound the pavement, but I am flying above the pavement in a sort of dance with the elements. While I was running in the St. George marathon, I was focused on running and finishing the race and went beyond anything I had done before. There was a time when as I was running and praying to be able to finish, I felt angels assisting me in the race. This was the ultimate connection between exercise, mind, and spirit. I am convinced that I would not have been able to have finished the race without this.

You do not have to be a prophet, a pro athlete, or a yoga master to be able to experience these connections. It is just a matter of knowing that these things are possible and you need to approach health in a different way. Instead of thinking that you need to lose weight and get healthier because when you look in a mirror you think you are fat, or you have a hard time doing things because you are overweight or out of shape, you need to think of health as something that is part of you just like your spirit is part of you and you need to exercise it with prayer, scripture study, and doing your callings in the church.

Habits

Most people would not be able to go more than a day or two without brushing their teeth, taking a shower, or texting on their cell phones, but they would not think twice about missing a few days reading their scriptures, skipping their exercise routine, or indulging in sweets. You need to first see health as developing healthy habits that will be part of your lifestyle just like brushing your teeth every day is.

It is the discipline of developing the habits which will help you to be more mindful of your health and start to live healthier. Many people follow programs because they start the process of these healthy habits and routines that direct people in the right direction. The problem as stated before is that these programs are someone else's programs and not yours. You need to do some research and develop your own program that will cause you to develop healthy habits that you will be able to follow the rest of your life, making modifications from time to time in order to be able to improve on it.

You need to get a notebook that you will be able to take notes on about some of the research you have collect and brainstorm some ideas about a program you can follow. This program needs to include your physical, mental, spiritual, social, financial, and environmental health. Do not make it so overwhelming that you are unable to get into the habit of following your program because it is too complex or too time consuming that you are unable to do it. Once you have come up with the blueprints for your own program then you should be able to come up with some ways in which you will be able to accomplish the program and make it apart of your lifestyle and a habit that will last the rest of your life. Keep the plan simple and easy to start so that you can make it a habit and then later you can add things to it. Remember line upon line and not to run faster than you are able.

If you are unable to follow your plan, and feel that it is too much, you need to rethink your plan and make some changes. It is important to start with the necessities in your plan. As an example the prophet has told us to read the scriptures every day, pray every day, and to do these things with our families as well. So this should be part of your plan, you can determine how long you read your scriptures and incorporate these things into other things you do. For instance I have often read my scriptures by listening to them on the way to work, or while I am jogging in the morning. You can multitask your health program to include many different things, and in terms of how it affects your health routine, it will enhance it and make it better if you are able to incorporate several other elements of health.

The prophets have also asked us to have family home evening, fulfill our callings, attend our meetings, attend the temple, and do family history work. Just the spiritual side of the health triangle can seem overwhelming, but remember Nephi's words that the Lord will give no commandment unless he has prepared away for us to accomplish the commandment. Also included in the commandments is the Word of Wisdom, and elements of physical health. We are commanded to eat right, sleep right, and to not be idle which includes not only exercise but work as well.

Start out by making a list of all of the essentials when it comes to all of these areas of health and then place them in some sort of routine or schedule to follow. Some of it has already been done for you like having family home evening on Monday night, and church meetings on Sunday. You might have scheduled exercising in the morning along with prayer and reading scriptures.

Diet should be just part of what you eat each day without any extra time involved with meals, except for a more thought up grocery list and meal preparation for healthier meals. By planning out your shopping list, you can just stick to it and not buy anything else and make the decision before hand that you are not going to buy any ice cream or doughnuts. If you stick to your shopping list and do not go shopping when you are hungry then you should do great in buy healthy food choices.

When it comes to social health you can just make it part of your normal life with the addition of being an active listener and paying attention to those around you looking for acts of charity or kindness to others. It doesn't take any more time to smile, say, "Hi," or do a small act of kindness to someone who needs it. You may need to reexamine how you treat your family and make adjustments to the amount of time you spend with your family and the things you do for your family.

Financial health can be done once a week in family council and is a matter of paying attention to the things you buy and watching your budget. With financial health you need to make a list of priorities that you follow first before looking making financial decisions. If your life is consumed with your finances and it is taking up too much time then there is something wrong.

Just like in anything in life if there is any aspect of your life that is taking too much of your time you are probably not using your time wisely and need to rethink the time you are spending in that area. There have been times in my life where I have spent too much time writing, exercising, and even too much time on spiritual activities. If something is affecting the other areas of your health because you are not doing other things.

It takes more than six weeks to develop a habit, so you need to stick with theme until you feel like you do not have to continue to motivate you into doing these things. You need to be diligent in following your routines and your program. Once you have developed these healthy habits you will be able to reflect on them and change them as necessary in order to make the proper modifications that will work for you.

Motivation

Motivation is the hardest part of health, the motivation to wake up early to go on a walk, or to continue to exercise day after day when you do not feel like it. You might think that you should start out with motivation when it comes to getting ready to follow a health program. But I have found that sometimes you just have to force yourself to do things and develop habits then the motivation will naturally come.

It is like gaining a testimony, you cannot just have a testimony first before actually living the gospel. Missionaries do not start out by saying you need to have a testimony of the gospel, they talk about other people like Joseph Smith, and teach the plan of salvation, challenge investigators to read the Book of Mormon, and to pray about it. It is the doing that brings about the testimony that these things are the real thing. Then once you have your testimony it is the testimony that compels or motivates you to go to church for three hours on Sunday and to pay your tithing, and do other things in the church.

The same thing applies to the motivation to exercise, eat right, and work on your social health. You need to follow your routines and your program, develop the habits, see the blessings you have, and then with this renewed testimony you can be motivated to continue your program and to seek to live a healthy life. Motivation should come from a deeper source one that is not based on pride or false assumptions. It should come from the joy and happiness you have when you exercise, when you do things for other, when you eat a healthy salad.

You should be motivated to exercise 30 plus minutes a day so that you are fit enough to go on hikes with your grandchildren, healthy enough to fulfill your family and church responsibilities. My main motivation when I exercise or eat right is my family. I pray, read the scriptures, and jog in the mornings because I want to be there for my daughter. I want to teach her the correct way to live, I also want her to be able to experience all that I have experienced. My secondary motivation is know how I feel when I do exercise, when I listen to other people and help others, and how I feel when I eat healthy foods. I might also be motivated to lose some weight or get in shape to hike up a mountain or complete in a race, but these things only come after my other motivations.

Including others

Successful health programs involve other people. You can do a lot alone to be healthy, and depending on your situation you might be doing a lot of it on your own. But most of us have families, friends, and coworkers who make up a majority of our lives, and to ignore them in our program would be foolish. Not only do you have to include the people in your life in your social health, but when it comes to finances, environment and spiritual health you need to include your family, friends, and in some cases your coworkers or people you go to school with.

Another powerful motivator is to have someone by your side with your program. It becomes a lot easier to get out of bed in the morning if you know that your neighbor down the street will be waiting for you at the park to jog a couple of miles, or you are taking yoga classes with your spouse who is going through the same things as you are. Some people naturally have people in their lives who exercise with them, share healthy cooking tips, and help to improve social health in their lives.

But there are others who despite their best efforts are unable to encourage their spouse or children to exercise with them or to do other healthy things with them. This becomes a major challenge in their overall health, because it will affect their social health and they will be less motivated to exercise especially when their spouse complains about them exercising too much, or criticizes them for trying to be healthy. Just like the journey you took to develop a program you can help your spouse, children, and friends do the same. You might even be fortunate to develop a program along with your spouse that you both can follow and experience things along the way together.

When you are about to do things with other people both of you will be able to motivate each other, share things with each other, and grow closer to each other. There is nothing more intimate that to be able to share your health with another person. I am often concerned when I see women or men out walking or jogging alone while there spouse is doing something else. Just like in the gospel if there is a part member family the family's spiritual health suffers.

If there is only one member of the family who is exercising then the family's physical health will suffer. I would prefer to live long with my family and my family doing physical things together with each other like hiking to the top of a mountain, than to watch helplessly on the sidelines as members of my family have health problems. It is so much better if families were healthy together just like how they go to church together and have family home evenings together.

Make it part of your life

Health should not be considered a separate part of your life, it should be your life. You should be thinking in terms of healthy living all of the time. When you go grocery shopping you should be looking to buy those things that are healthy for you and your family and not even considering buying things that are not. Each day you should be thinking about ways to exercise, to incorporate reading your scriptures and praying.

Many people do this already in some form or another. I wake up early every morning and exercise, and have done this every since I was in high school. Other people read so many pages or for so long in the their scriptures each morning or night regardless of what day it is or where they are even when they are on vacation. Once you have made health part of your life, then you do not have to make such an effort to make health as a habit, because it will be part of you.

You will find that your desires will shift and instead of wanting to watch a late night movie, and sleep in on Saturday. You desire to get to bed early so that you can wake up and get to the trailhead early in the morning to climb a mountain you have been thinking about. The taste of food will change and you will find pop, and sweets disgusting, and fruits and vegetables tasty. Your senses will be heightened to the point where you will be able to smell the trees, taste the water vapor in the air before it rains, and hear the clocks in your house ticking down the seconds.

Everything in your life will seem more real to you and more vibrant. You will no longer feel depressed or sad, but joyful to greet every day. Each challenge will be welcomed into your life as a learning experience. You will no longer have to think about the future and worry about what will happen tomorrow, the next week, or the next year because you are comfortable at what you are accomplishing in the present and are confident that what you are doing today will have a positive influence on the future.

The aches and pains of the past will be replaced with an occasional soreness from time to time. You will be able to go years without getting sick and when you do start to feel a sore throat coming or a change in your health you will be able to attach it full force and prevent it from getting full blown. A cold that normally would last eight days with an altering running and stuffy nose, aches and pains, chills, and coughing will only last about a day with some aches and pains, a slight stuffy nose and a little sneezing and coughing, but in a day or two it is all gone and you are back to normal.

The relationships in your life will be great with close friendships and a closeness in your family that you could only wish for in the next life. You will be able to communicate your feelings to others and understand what other people are saying to you without having miscommunication take place. You are no longer afraid to talk to people, because you know that they will not get upset with you when you talk to them.

All aspects of your life improves including your job where it is less stressful, you enjoy working with other people at your job, and you feel great at the end of the day when you come home. Every part of your life is filled with joy and excitement that was missing before. Life becomes your own part of heaven on earth and you find yourself wanting to share it with others and have a bit of sadness in your heart when other people have a hard time changing their life for the better.

Balance and Harmony

As in all things there needs to be a balance or a sense of harmony that is established when it comes to health. There are times in your life that you will be out of balance in your health because of illness, accident, or injury. You may also be going through a social crisis like a divorce or a spiritual crisis where you might have committed a sin. You might even be out of harmony because you are spending too much time on one aspect of your health while ignoring the others. It is not uncommon to neglect your family because you are spending too much time on your church callings, or you might be spending too much time of recreational pursuits like fishing, camping, or hiking that you miss church, or you exercise too much and your social life suffers.

It is hard for a person to keep their life in balance when they are training for the Olympics, or working towards a Ph.D. Life tends to change our priorities from time to time with the change of jobs, relationships, and church callings. One moment you might be working a job that goes from 9 to 5 the next working graveyard. You might have a goal to run a marathon and have to spend an extra two hours a day exercising. A person may be called to be the Bishop of your ward or Stake President, Relief Society president or Primary President. All of these things will shift the harmony of your life and you have to change things in order to adapt. This means that you might have to change your sleeping pattern, how much time you exercise, or move to another area and leave behind friends you have made to make new friends where you move to.

Achieving balance and harmony in your life when it comes to health is crucial, and it can be done given your lifestyle and modified according to changes in your life and changes in your goal. If you have set a goal to run in a marathon you simply change the amount of time you spend on other exercises and add it to running so that you can get in shape as far as running is concerned. At one point in my life I had a goal to compete in power lifting so I spent a lot of time in the gym weight lifting. Then once I competed in a competition, I wanted to run a marathon, so I changed my workouts into doing more running, and biking. Now I am not so concerned with too much endurance or strength but a more moderate level of each with more emphasis on Tai Chi and Yoga which I believe will carry me through till my death.

I know through a lot of struggles in my life that getting out of harmony is not a good thing. There have been times I have gotten burned out in exercise and I started to get sick and loss strength instead of maintaining or gaining it. The only solution I could do was not to exercise so much, and once I slowed down and started to be a less fanatical with my exercise I was able to gain control of my body and life again.

There is no way of telling how you can have balance or harmony in your life. You have to find that out for yourself. You may prefer to so more spiritual things in your life, more social, or more in terms of finance. Someone else might be more into being an athlete and will exercise more and watch their diet more than you do. It is a personal preference and requires you to find out what your goals are and how you feel as you implement things in your life.

You should start to recognize when you are going out of harmony in your life when your relationships suffer, or you have a hard time concentrating. You might find yourself fatigued and exhausted easily. If your health starts to change for the worse it might because the balance in your life has altered to the point that it is causing some problems in your life.

It is important to restore the balance and harmony in your life so that you can continue to life a healthy life and be able to enjoy life. It is not how long you live that matters, it is the quality of your life that matters the most. If you only live to be 35 years old and your life is filled with love, joy, and excitement then you have lived a great life, compared to someone who lives to be a 100 years old and just sits on the couch wasting 50 years of their life being depressed and having all kinds of small illnesses that plague and torture them.

In achieving a balance in your life, you need to develop a plan or program that incorporates all of the major elements of health discusses in this book. Adjust it according to your lifestyle and the goals you have for yourself, and reexamine it from time to time making the necessary adjustments along the way.

Once you have achieved harmony in your life with your health and have developed your habits, you will be able to let go on of the restraints of being strict in your routines and rely more on the spirit and where life will take you. The idea would be to life your life in harmony with the spirit and with your health. This means that one week you might spend a week in the mountains, the next week you are learning to play the piano, and another week you are with your parents whose health is failing.

The key to having a healthy life is achieving this level of harmony where you do not have to worry, and you have no more fear, your faith is what brings you high upon the mountains of your health. The only task from then on would be to maintain the balance and harmony in your life in all aspects of health. You then will be able to live a healthy happy life that extends to your family and friends as well as the church and those you have in contact with in the church.

Record Keeping

Some people are very organized and are able to keep detailed records of their workouts, what they eat, and how they interact with others. But record keeping can be time consuming and tedious. It is important to keep some form of record in order to see what you have done and if there are any changes you need to make in order to improve your life.

It could be something as simple as keeping a reflective journal of your experiences in health. This is where you would record what you did and your personal feelings about what is going on in your life. You will be able to see what you have done and compare it from week to week and to be able to reflect on it and use it as a tool to help you modify your workout, and the things you do in your life for health. A journal could be recorded in once a week and you can write in the things you did that week and think about the changes you can make for the next week. You can keep one journal or several depending on how detailed you want to be. For instance you can keep a journal on exercising, a journal on diet, and a journal on social interactions. You may even wish to keep a separate record of your financial transactions.

If you prefer to be more specific and detailed when it comes to all the areas of your health you can keep a detailed log entry for all of the things you do. This can be time consuming, but it will give you a better more accurate picture of what you are able to accomplish and give you enough information for you to be able to alter your routines and actions for the next week or month that you need to change.

I would suggest that you try both and see what works best for you. If you are into technology you can simply keep your journal on your electronic device or online. You might even have a program that you have on computer that you like to keep track of what you are doing. There are a lot of financial programs you can get that will help you manage your finances that are worth looking into.

It might seem silly to keep track of your conversations or interactions with other people, but it will help you to see how you handled the situation and what you could do the next time you were in that situation. You can record your feelings when someone said something to you and use that to help you in your prayers for the day. You are able to reflect upon and repent of sins you might have committed during the day.

Think of the record keeping part of health as just another element of your health. It can be very therapeutic to your mental and social health and will help your improve your physical health and even your spiritual health as you are able to listen to the spirit more through your pondering and be able to work on improving your health. You should at least do some recording at least once a week, but doing it once a day can also be very beneficial to you, because it gives you a change to look at your day and a change to be able to change a bad habit as you work on it from day to day.

To Do List

1. Make health part of every aspect of your life.
2. Seek balance and harmony in your health and your life not overdoing it in any area of your health.
3. Record what you do as regards to your health so that you will be able to examine it and alter it according to the intensions of the commander.
4. Look at the things that motivate you deep down and allow them to continue to motivate you on your journey of health
5. Develop healthy habits that will last you a lifetime.
6. Include others in your quest to be healthy especially members of your family and friends.
7. Develop a program that is based on your lifestyle and goals.
8. Continue to do research on health and healthy practices.
9. Learn to love what you do and enjoy life.
10. Pay attention to the blessing you receive and show gratitude to the Lord and others.

Chapter Ten: The Cure

"… I am the way, the truth, and the life:…" (John 14:7)

Billions of people worldwide suffer through poverty going to bed hungry and not knowing when or where they will get their next meal. People around the world watch as members of their family die from all manner of diseases. Almost everyone at one time or another goes through a period of depression and spiritual death where they are separated from God and the Spirit of the Lord.

We spend trillions of dollars each year in search for an end to starvation, war, disease, and making us able to live longer. Brilliant scientist are searching of the cure to these things, and many religious leaders are claiming that they are the way to salvation. Movies give stories of struggle and death with the hope of overcoming death and having the hero vanquish the foe who is bent on the destruction of the world.

The truth of this is that we already know the cure, and we already know what is going to happen to us after we die. We also know that we can see those who have died again and be with them through eternity. The knowing can comfort us and bring us joy through this life. Yet despite the knowledge of the cure and the idea that we will live forever and see our loved ones again still causes people to become distraught and depressed, and many people continue to exhibit destructive behavior.

It is through the temptations of Satan and his persuasiveness that causes us to doubt our knowledge of the afterlife, and the covenants we have made that have promises and blessing attached to them. We have to be reminded each day about who we are and where we will be going in order to maintain our faith and to be able to devote ourselves to a healthy life.

Satan's plan is to be able to drag people down with him and be just as miserable as he is. He persuades people to follow him according to the promise of temporary desires and passions that may give us temporary satisfaction and enjoyment, but in the long run are destructive in nature to our health. He might say that exercise is too hard and you do not need to do it. He would say that life is short and you should just enjoy it by drinking alcohol, smoking cigarettes, and using drugs. He may tell you that marriage is old fashioned and you should live together with other people first to see if the relationship would work out, and it is okay if the relationship doesn't work out, because you can always try out a relationship with someone else. There is no need for commitment, and you are number one. You should do everything to get a head in life even if it means that you have to hurt other people. There is only one winner in a race and it ought to be you. You have to fight to get the promotion at work and if you have to do something that is not ethical at the time it is okay, because you will be able to at least get your promotion.

The temptations might be something as simple as a thought or idea about something and this suddenly starts to consume you until you start to do what you were thinking. Everything has its opposites, so if God wants you to be healthy in all of the aspects of your life. Satan wants you to be unhealthy. Every unhealthy thing in life is from Satan and every healthy thing in life is from God. Seek to be healthy and you go closer to good, if you seek to be unhealthy you are drawing yourself further away from God.

Satan will do everything in his power to make you miserable and to prevent you from doing your church callings and other things in life. This is easily done if you are unhealthy, so strive to be healthy so that you can be happy, do what the Lord has asked of you, and are able to help others. Do not fall into the trap of the world of waiting until something is wrong and then attempting to fix it. Do not wait until you are sick and then have to see the doctor. Take the necessary steps to better health right now while you can and not wait until you are in a hospital. I have seen a lot of family and friends who do nothing for their health and then when they get sick they complain about getting sick and go to the doctor to get medicine to get them better, only they have to suffer the entire time.

The Cure is Prevention

Let me tell you a secret to the cure of cancer, heart disease, diabetes, Alzheimer's, depression, and many other illnesses. It is not a secret and almost everyone knows it, but it is so simple that many people do not even take advantage of it until it is too late and they die from one of these illnesses. Just like the children of Israel who only had to look up and see the serpent on the staff to be healed from the snake bites, we only have to follow this simple rule.

It is through the gospel we learn of this and it is also common sense among those who practice this. We can say that it is living a Christ like life, obeying the commandment of which the greatest is to love God and the second is to love our neighbor. In living the Word of Wisdom is promises us good health. If you look into the scriptures and the council of modern prophets you will know that living the gospel and other healthy standards you will be able to prevent these terrible diseases.

It is only through prevention you are able to cure or prevent terrible disease to infect others, and it is the same preventative practices that will help to cure people as they have the disease. There have been several people who when upon learning they have cancer or heart disease reverse their lifestyle and start to live a life they should have been living before and it has reversed their life just like how someone can repent of their sins, a person can repent of

195

their poor health habits and transform them into healthy people.

There are those who live healthy lives and still get sick and die, but this is rare exceptions. Even these people who do get cancer or have heart attacks are able to handle it with a positive attitude and many of them are able to overcome the challenge or to be able to die with dignity. Those who are healthy and suddenly are taken by cancer or some other accident or illness are able to overcome it or even are taken quickly like they were called home. But those who practice unhealthy lifestyles often suffer for years with poor health and their deaths are terrible.

Exercise and living healthy can prevent so many illnesses that there is no wonder drug that can even compare to it. There is nothing that can compare to good wholesome exercise and a healthy diet when it comes to preventing illness. If everyone were to just exercise and eat healthy on a regular basis cancer, heart disease, and diabetes would be cut by more than half in ten years. There would be billions of dollars that would be saved each year in medical expenses. It would completely transform society where people would be happy and instead of trying to compete with others people would be helping each other. There would be no need for the government to help people out because they would be able to take care of themselves.

The countless birth defects and genetic disorders would start to fall and there would be healthier babies born and the cost of emergency care for infants would go way down. If only people would work on the elements of health discussed in this book we would solve many of the ills of society such as poverty, poor health, violence, and lack of moral fiber. It is something that can be done and it can be done without too much cost to either the government, businesses, or the public.

The resistance to this would be by businesses that profit from the ill health of others such as the pharmaceutical companies, hospitals, and those who sale tobacco, alcohol, and illegal substances. Then there would be those individuals who are convinced that they have the right to destroy their health and the health of others. Americans get a sense that freedom means that they are able to do what they want to even when it comes to hurting themselves and others. They think that they have the right to do things regardless of the consequences.

So the simplest way to cure disease is to prevent it. Just like the simple act of looking at the serpent for the Children of Israel, we just have to live a healthy life through exercise, eating healthy, having enough sleep, good hygiene, having good posture, and breathing right. Healthy living also includes the spiritual things we do like attending church, the temple, reading scriptures, and prayer. It is communicating effectively with others, having integrity and charity toward others. Healthy living is planning out a budget and sticking with it. You can be healthy by keeping the air you breathe and the water you drink clean. Being healthy also means keeping your mind sharp through reading, and study of new things.

It might seem a daunting task to have to do all of these things in order to be healthy and to be able to prevent the illness. Many people choose to take their chances and get sick rather than to put forth the effort to be healthy. Just like those who would rather choose to die from the snake bite than to look up at the serpent on the pole. I would be lying if I said that it didn't take a lot of effort to live a healthy life, but it is also easy once you realize that it is just part of your life anyway, and that by being healthy it frees up all of the time you would have spent doing unhealthy activities, and being sick. Also I would rather put forth the effort in order to be happy than to sit around and wallow in suffering and sadness.

I find that life is so much more enjoyable when I am engaged in a good cause, and my health is one of the best causes I can think of and that of the health of others I know. The benefits completely out way the effort that is involved in it, and the investment is huge when it comes to your health. Imagine buying an old beat up house that needs a lot of work in it. You spend a lot of your own time and money into making the house look nice. It takes you a year or two before it is finished. When you are finished, you find that you can sell the house for more than twice you paid for it. All of the time and money you spent on it suddenly becomes worth it. While during the time you were fixing it up you doubted if it would be worth it and feared that you would lose money on the deal.

  The same applies to your health. While you are working on being healthy it might seem hard work and you are not sure you will get your investment back on the deal. It will take several months or years before you will realize all of the benefits you are receiving by your efforts. The prevention suddenly becomes the cure. This is often overlooked because you have a different perspective when you do get sick as opposed to when you do not get sick. When you do get sick, you definitely want to get better and not be sick anymore, but when you are healthy getting sick doesn't have much of an impact because you have not experienced what it is like.

  If we would just take all of the resources we use to finding cures into the prevention part of health we would be able to do amazing things, and not just look at one area of health, but all areas of health including spiritual. Not only does society focus on treatment of the illness and finding the cure, it often ignores the other aspects of health. When was the last time you heard your doctor ask you if you have been saying your daily prayers or been reading your scriptures as part of your health plan? It is not often a doctor will suggest a priesthood blessing or give advice for people to treat their spouses better.

The medical community is so diversified with specialist in every field that it is often a nightmare to figure out what is wrong with you and then the bill from seeing all of those specialist practically kills you when you get it. It isn't any wonder that people who get sick and have huge medical bills continue to have health problems, because of the stress of having to pay for the bills. There is also the atmosphere of many hospitals where people are coming in and out of your room asking you all these questions like they are interrogating you and taking all of these tests that seem to be more routine than necessary. I cannot imagine getting better in a hospital, but getting worse because of the atmosphere and the stress involved with being in a hospital.

This is why people get better faster the sooner they can come home from the hospital and be in the loving care of their family and friends. I have yet to experience a medical system whose business is making people better as a person helping the person to be work on their entire health. I have heard of such places, but am not sure that these places include spiritual and financial health. I know that there are specialized spas where you can get massages, acupuncture, and they will help you lose weight and eat right as well as exercise, but they lack the spiritual side of things unless it is the Eastern religious thought found in Yoga and Buddhism. These places also tend to be very expensive which puts stress on the person's financial health.

I believe that if medical centers where to consolidate all of the specialists and that a patient was treated through their entire health and not just physically, and they were treated more as a member of the family, the patients would get better faster, enjoy the experience so much more. Medical centers should also be preventative centers where people can go to get routine exams, tests, access to a gym, and access to other areas of health that are often reserved for special treatment centers such as herbal medicine, acupuncture, massage, and meditation.

Being Your Own Personal Trainer and Doctor

Today you need to be your own personal trainer and doctor in order to have better access to your health and to save money on what can be a very expensive process of being healthy. Once you have started to take an interest in your health and become more aware of your body, mind and spirit you will be able to understand what is happening to your health better than any doctor or personal trainer can. You are the only one who can know what your body is telling you when you go out for a job and you feel like you are overdoing it, or when you are slacking off and need to put in an extra mile.

You should be able to tell when you are getting depressed, you are eating things you should not eat, you are spending too much money on things you do not need, and you have not been faithful in saying your prayers or reading your scriptures. No expert can tell you what is happening in your life better than you can. You just have to listen to your body, your mind, your spirit, and examine all other aspects of your health and determine what you need to do to make your health in harmony with your life.

A personal trainer and doctor would first have you go through a physical exam and have you go through a series of tests to determine where you are in terms of your health. One thing they may not do is to determine what your mental and spiritual health is, and will not consider your financial well being or your environment and your social health. This is why it is important for you to take charge, because you can look at these other areas to determine where you are. If you are doing great physically exercising, getting enough sleep, eating right, and have good hygiene then you do not have to spend a lot of time in that area of your health, but you might find that you have not been to church in several weeks, haven't been praying or reading your scriptures. Then you simply have to make a record of those things you need to do and start to do them.

Once the personal trainer has determined where you are in terms of your physical health he would then ask you about some goals you want to accomplish which is generally in terms of losing weight, getting stronger, and having more energy and based on those goals he would put together a routine in order for you to accomplish those goals. Then he would teach you how to do it, encourage you to stick with the program, and monitor your progress making changes from time to time. The problem is that the personal trainer and your doctor do not have the whole picture of your health, and may not know what you are thinking, feelings, or truly wanting to happen with your fitness routine. You need to develop your own routine and stick with it by making it part of your life.

The same goes with all the other areas of your health. You can spend thousands of dollars in hiring a personal trainer and be supervised by a doctor, and then do the same with a psychologist for your mental health, a sociologist for your social health, a financial consultant for your financial health, and spending time with your bishop on your spiritual health. You can even consult someone on feng shui and a gardener for your yard. In some of these areas you might need extra advice or help from an expert, but it would be madness to have to spend a lot of money seeing a lot of people who may or may not help you.

It is hard to say what is best for a person, but the best way to take charge of your health is for you to become the expert on your own health and to study and learn about physical, mental, social, financial, environmental, and spiritual health. Once you are able to do this then the rest is a piece of cake. It is just a matter of doing it, and by working on this you will be able to help others around you, and you might even find a career that you are interest in. By focusing on your health and working through these things you will be able to have a more complete experience.

Many people fail to get in shape and be healthy, because they either expect a magic pill, routine, or other personal such as a personal trainer to do it for them. Once they realize that it is a lot of work and they have to put in a lot of time and effort they give up on the idea of being healthy. Yet once they have gone through all of the hard work to learn more about health and to start doing it in their lives they are more committed to being healthy. I did not get into running until I devoted a year of my life training for a marathon, and once I did that I have been devoted to running ever since. Every time I take the time and effort to do something, I appreciate it more and I am more committed to it.

It is advisable to see a doctor and at least go through a complete physical when starting a fitness program, and you should get an exam at least once a year, just like you should see your dentist at least twice a year. A physical exam will also help you to check if there are any concerns to have to be aware of such as high blood pressure. It will also be a set point that you can check in a year to see if you are healthier than you were the year before. You may already have a health concern like diabetes that you should have monitored by a doctor especially as you change your lifestyle.

When you are starting a program and are starting to change your lifestyle, be patient and do not get over zealous, many people overdue it at first, because they are excited about getting in shape and losing weight. The problem is that there can be a lot of challenges when you start to overdue it. You can burn yourself out causing your body and mind to be more fatigued and exhausted than you have been before. You could get injured pushing your body more than it can take, and you could start to get sick because your body is not used to the increase in fitness level.

Take things slowly, and be patient with your health it will not come over night and it might be weeks, or months before you see results and you can start to accomplish your goals. If you do have a goal to run in a marathon or complete in some event, it is important to leave enough training time to accomplish this, do not wait to the last few months to train for something that takes six months or longer to train for. Listen to your body, your mind, and your spirit to determine just how much you can push yourself. You do want to push yourself a little so that you will be able to see some improvement, but you need not be like an Olympic athlete who trains six or more hours a day.

Be the Cure

Be the cure to what illness you might have. If you are depressed make it a point to exercise, eat right, get the right amount of sleep and not sleep longer than is needful, have positive thoughts, read your scriptures, pray, attend meetings, and do what you can to distress your life. Depression is often the result of a combination of things. You might be depressed because you feel lonely, you are out of shape, and you have credit card debt. I order to cure your depression you need to get out of debt, start getting in shape, make an effort to see people, and get your health back in balance with your life.

If you have high blood pressure and are overweight you can exercise more, eat less, and make sure that all of the other area of your health are in line with your life. You will slowly lose weight, and your health will return to harmony with your life, and you can lower your blood pressure to the point that you will not have to take blood pressure medication. Many people can get off of medications and other treatment if they were to just become healthy by their own right. It is important, however to consult with your doctor about your plans and to be cautious when working on eliminating medications from your life. Some medications if taken away may cause a life threatening condition, and you may not understand what the medication is doing for you.

You can take charge of your life and of your health all areas of your health. This will help you to be able to do so much more for yourself and others as you can have more freedom in your life. The harder you work on being healthy the more you are able to accomplish in your life overall. Just think if you are able to have financial freedom having no debts, you are physically able to hike up to the top of mountains, ride a mountain bike in Moab, and you have enough faith in yourself that you can talk to others about ideas and concerns you have about things at work, at home, and in the community. There would be nothing you would not be able to do given you are healthy in all areas of your health.

There will be a lot of challenges that you will have to face in regards to your health. Especially when you look at all of the areas of your health, you might find that you will be facing challenges on a daily basis with your health. This will be part of the process of being healthy. You just have to take charge and restore the balance when one area of your health suffers. As an example your car might break down and you will have to buy another one, which would put you in debt. But as you work through it you are able to buy a used car for less and come up with a plan to be able to pay off the car in only a short period of time.

Satan and his followers will continue to place challenges in your path and work towards making you discouraged and distraught when it comes to working on your health and attempting to make it sustainable. Just remember that Satan wants you to be miserable and the best way to do this is to get you to be unhealthy. I am the happiest when my health is in harmony with my life and I consider myself healthy. If I am unhealthy then I grow increasingly restless and depressed. Do not get discouraged, because you can expect to have set backs and challenges when it comes to your health and you will find that these things are often temporary and in the end if you do not give up you will be able to experience the blessings of being healthy.

Giving Up

The single worst thing you can do in your life would be to give up. To stop working on being healthy and call it quits. People who give up become unhealthy and lose all of the blessings that would come from being healthy. Giving up could meant that you decide you no longer want to go to church, and you stop reading your scriptures and praying. You might still exercise and eat right, but there will be a void in your life and you will not be able to receive the blessings of the church and the fellowship of the saints as well as future consequences of allowing your spiritual health to suffer.

You might be a faithful member of the church and follow everything except that you have a bad habit of eating too much and you find exercise too much work for you, so you decide not to worry about exercising anymore. Your spiritual side may be in tack, but you start to suffer from a series of minor physical illnesses that progress into full blown cancer, heart disease, diabetes, or other health conditions.

It is important not to give up, make a commitment to be healthy and to stick with it as you make it part of your life. The consequences of giving up are just too great to even consider. If things seem to be too overwhelming when it comes to exercise, then scale back and reexamine your routine. It might be that you are exercising too much, and that you need to go at a slower pace when it comes to exercise. But do not give up completely on exercise or any other part of your health.

You may find it too hard to read a chapter a day in the Book of Mormon, or find the time to be able to read. So then you can listen to the Book of Mormon on audio book format while you exercise or do house chores, or instead of a chapter a day it is a page a day, or a half a page a day. Just do not give up reading your scriptures.

If you give up you are giving in to Satan, he knows that by giving up you are allowing him to take charge of your life, instead of you taking charge of your life, and allowing the Holy Ghost to guide you. It is this guidance that is essential when it comes to your health. By keeping in tune and striving to be healthy, the Holy Ghost and the atonement of Christ will assisted and comfort you in your quest to be healthy. The main purpose and mission of the Godhead is to have you return to the Father and to achieve exaltation. Your Heavenly Father wants you to be happy and he knows that in order to be happy you need to be healthy as well. It is up to you to do your part and ponder the things you need to do to be healthy and then to do them. With the Lord's help and with a little determination you will be able to be healthy and to be able to do amazing things in your life.

Eternal Health

Now that you have read this book and have started on your journey to have better health in your life. You need to start thinking about health in terms of eternity. All things are eternal including health. You might not carry into the next life financial health or even environmental health, but these things help you to gain more discipline and help you to gain more control over other area of health. Financially you learn not to be envious or greedy, and look more at using money for necessities and in helping those who need help. In the millennium and the spirit world there is no need for money, but the concept of helping others and overcoming greed will still exist.

The environment will also be a little different, but environmental health will help us to have greater respect for the environment and it will help us to see the true beauty of life. Some day we may be able to create our own world and in them the beauty at which we have seen here in this world.

Our social relations on this earth are eternal and will be confirmed upon our righteousness and being sealed together as families in the temple. Eternal families will lead our existence in the afterlife and will be the catalyst for our eternal progression. So the relationships we develop on this earth are in good measure the relationships we will have for eternity. It is this fact that drives most of us to do the things we do on this earth. If it wasn't for eternal relations then everything would be for not. Those you do not believe in eternal relations and the departure of death are unable to glimpse eternity and the joy one receives at being with a loved one throughout eternity. Many people hope that they will be able to see those they love when they die, but do not know how this will take place.

When we look at our relations we are building eternal ones. This means that we are looking beyond death and a temporary partnership that will end at death. When you work on your social health you need to look in terms of eternal relationships and focus on those things that will help this. If you have bad habits when it comes to respect, or choosing to be nice to only certain people with a refusal to help others then you will lose this eternal focus. This is where the teachings of Jesus comes in where he wanted all people to love their enemies, their neighbors and to take care of the sick and afflicted.

Physical health might be another area that might be hard to transfer to the eternal perspective. Once we have perfected resurrected bodies we will not have to worry about illness, pain, or any other physical malady. But there is something about our bodies that has an eternal perspective on things, and it is one thing that separates us from Satan and his followers is that we have a body. You might think that is doesn't matter how bad you treat your body in this life because you will get a resurrected body in the next. But there is an eternal bond between the body and the spirit that is only broken momentarily when the spirit leaves the body at death.

The body is what gives us a lot of temptations of the flesh in this life that we have to overcome. How we treat our bodies in this life has an influence on our spirit and it does talk about different resurrections of people. There is the celestial resurrection which will take place on the morning of the first resurrection and those who are not so righteous will be resurrected after those on the morning of the first. Those resurrected on the afternoon of the first day will receive the resurrection of those going to the terrestrial kingdom. The second day will consist of those in the telestial kingdom and those who were cast off into outer darkness. The glory of our bodies will be given to us according to which kingdom we enter. So each of our bodies will be different, and part of this is in condition to how we treat our bodies because they are considered temples of God and this will relate to our spiritual health.

This is one reason why modern prophets have cautioned against tattoos, piercings and other things that damage the body or alter its appearance. We will have eternal bodies and hey are temples of God and we need to start treating them as such. It can be difficult at time to conceive that how we treat our bodies will affect our eternal progression, but it does matter, or the prophets would not have said anything.

"Wherefore, they are bodies terrestrial, and not bodies celestial, and differ in glory as the moon differs from the sun. And again, we saw the glory of the telestial, which glory is that of the lesser, even as the glory of the stars differs from that of the glory of the moon in the firmament." (D&C 76:78, 81)

Mental health is something you can see will continue on with you through your thoughts, emotions, and ideas. It is the very thoughts that come to your mind that cause you to take action and it is the intent of your heart that you will be judged. If a man were to deceive people with much flattery and to win people over to his side, but his intent or thoughts are to just hurt others his thoughts will come back on him and he will be judged by them.

"Yea, and cry unto God for all thy support; yea let all thy doings be unto the lord, and withersoever thou goest let it be in the Lord; yea , let all thy thoughts be directed unto the Lord; yea, let the afflections of thy heart be placed upon the Lord forever." (Alma 37:36)

I am certain that someone who dies with evil intentions heart and in his mind that he will not be able to go into the celestial kingdom. It doesn't mean that we cannot repent of our ways and to clean up our thoughts so that we will be forgiven and then be able to return to Heavenly Father. If you know that your thoughts will be reviewed at judgment day and your intent will be shown you will have a different perspective on eternal mental health.

Jesus set the standard when he told the people that it is a sin to look after a woman and lust after her and a man has committed adultery in his heart. We have to look at how our thoughts will affect our eternal progress. This is why it is important not to watch rated "R," movies, programming that will cause us to have unhealthy thoughts.

This might be images from the internet, or phone. It may not be the deeds that we do in the last days that will condemn us but our thoughts that will condemn us.

Spiritual health is much easier to put into the context of eternity. All things spiritual are eternal this includes the covenants we make at baptism and at the temple. Having access to the atonement in our lives will help us to grow closer to the Savior and his teachings which are eternal teaching that will help us to achieve our eternal goals. Spiritual health is the foundation of health and of eternity, this is why it was first in this book for a healthy practice, and the last thing in the book. If we are to seek spiritual health then all other practices of health will fall in line. It must be seen in terms of eternity and how we can continue to do what we do for eternity.

To Do List

1. Focus on prevention with being healthy and not wait to treat the illness.
2. Be your own personal trainer and take charge of your health.
3. Assess your overall health and get a physical from a doctor to see where you are and to check to see if there are any concerns.
4. Know that you will have many challenges in all of the areas of your health and you need to just concentrate on overcoming them.
5. Never give up, be courageous and have faith in yourself that you will be able to become healthy.
6. Develop a network of people you can rely on to help you with your health. This could include your doctor, bishop, neighbor, and family. It might also include people from work or people you know who are able to help you when it comes to health.
7. Seek help from the Lord through prayer and fasting to help you in developing a health program of your own and sticking with this program.
8. Find ways to motivate you to continue with your program, this might involve making short and long term goals, and giving yourself small rewards for your effort. Beware of giving yourself unhealthy rewards for being healthy like going out to an all you can eat restaurant because you were able to lose five pounds during the week, or taking two weeks off after being able to exercise for six months.
9. Be persistent and diligent at sticking with your program, the benefits of your work will not be seen until after the trial of your faith and after you have vanquished all of your foes.
10. Share your success with others and encourage other people you know to be healthy.

Appendix A

Spiritual Checklist

Name: _____   Date: _____

Goal:

Activities that the prophets said that you need to do on a daily basis.	Activities prophets have said you need to do each week.	Activities prophets have said you should do on a monthly basis.
Personal Prayers: Family Prayers:	Attend church meetings:	Attend the temple:
Personal Scripture Study: Family Scripture Study:	Fulfill church callings:	Do home/visiting teaching:
Dinner as a family:	Have Family Home Evening:	
	Write in your journal: Hold Family Council:	

Appendix B

Mental Checklist

Name: _____ Date: _____
Goal:

Mental Exercise on a daily basis	Mental Exercise you can do on a weekly basis	Mental Exercises you can do on a monthly basis
Repeat memorized quotes, scriptures:		
Read books some of which you can listen to in audio book format:		

Appendix C

Physical Checklist

Name: _____Date: _____
Goal:

Daily activities	Weekly activities	Monthly activities
Sleep around 8 hours going to be and waking up at the same time:		
Eating healthy foods with emphasis on fruits and vegetables and whole grains:		
Exercise including endurance, strength, and flexibility exercises:		
Practice good hygiene habits of brushing teeth, taking shower, and washing hands:		

Appendix D

Social Health

Name: _____   Date: _____
Goal:

Daily Activities	Weekly Activities	Monthly Activities
Be an active listener excited about everything people say:		
Look for the opportunity to do something kind:		

Appendix E

Environmental Checklist

Name: _____   Date: _____
Goal:

Daily Activities	Weekly Activities	Monthly Activities

Appendix F

Financial Checklist

Name: _____   Date: _____
Goal:

Daily Activities	Weekly Activities	Monthly Activities

Appendix G

Health Circle

Write those things you care about the most in your health circle.

www.ingramcontent.com/pod-product-compliance
Lightning Source LLC
Chambersburg PA
CBHW071341280526
45787CB00001B/175